The Other
Child

A Book for Parents and Laymen

THE OTHER CHILD

The Brain-Injured Child

Richard S. Lewis

Alfred A. Strauss

Laura E. Lehtinen

Second Revised and Enlarged Edition

Grune & Stratton • New York and London

Library of Congress Catalog No. 60-6019

First Edition
Copyright © 1951 and
Second Edition
Copyright © 1960 by
GRUNE & STRATTON, INC.
381 Park Avenue South
New York, N.Y. 10016

Second Edition:
First printing, March 1960
Second printing, February 1963
Third printing, February 1966

Printed in U.S.A. (G-B)

Contents

Dedication

Alfred A. Strauss, 1897-1957

Alfred A. Strauss, internationally known authority on the education and rehabilitation of brain-injured children, died at Michael Reese Hospital in Chicago, October 27, 1957. He was 60. He was born in Karlsruhe, Germany, May 29, 1897.

Dr. Strauss was President and Co-founder of The Cove Schools of Racine, Wisconsin and Evanston, Illinois. He had served as consultant to the Division of Special Education, Illinois Office of Public Instruction, and as special lecturer at Wayne University, Detroit and the Milwaukee State Teachers College, Milwaukee.

At the time of his death, Dr. Strauss was engaged in research in linguistics and aphasia. His pioneering work in educational rehabilitation of the brain-injured child with disturbances in perception and concept formation had won wide acceptance among educators, psychiatrists and psychologists.

Much of his interest was directed toward developing teaching methods which took into account the perceptual and conceptual disabilities of children whose brain functioning had been altered by injury.

The methods of teaching developed by Dr. Strauss and his associates have been applied successfully in special classes for children with disturbances in perception and concept formation in the Joliet, Illinois public school system and in Macon, Georgia.

Dr. Strauss received his medical degree from the University of Heidelberg in 1922. After five years of special training in psychiatry and neurology, he entered private practice and worked at the same time as research associate at the University Psychiatric Clinic in Heidelberg.

In 1930 he was appointed Director of the Outpatient Department of the University's Psychiatric and Neurological Clinic and became at the same time Associate Professor (Privatdozent) of Neuropsychiatry. He also was Child Welfare Consultant to the City of Heidelberg, its School Board and its Municipal Children's Home.

With the first rumblings of Hitler, Dr. Strauss left Germany. He was invited to Spain where he became, in 1933, visiting professor at the University of Barcelona and helped to establish the first public child guidance clinic. He also founded the first private child guidance clinic in Barcelona. Dr. Strauss left Spain at the outbreak of the Civil War.

He then came to the United States in 1937 to join the staff of the Wayne County Training School at Northville, Michigan, as a research psychiatrist. After becoming a naturalized citizen in 1943, he was appointed Director of Child Care of this institution.

Dr. Strauss held this post until 1946 when he resigned because of illness. In 1947, he founded The Cove Schools at Racine as a residential school for brain-injured children. The Evanston day unit was established in 1950.

In his early years in the United States Dr. Strauss devoted his attention to developing a number of qualitative tests for the diagnosis of brain injury in children. The psychological examination of problem children has been greatly and lastingly enriched by the tests as psychological tools as well as by the description of the clinical picture of the behavior and response characteristics of the brain-injured child. The result has been a distinct refinement in the differential diagnosis of the brain-injured, neurotic and psychotic child.

One of Dr. Strauss' major contributions was the demonstration of differences in mental organization between the brain-injured mentally retarded (exogenous) child and the familial mentally retarded (endogenous) child. Through these researches the long-held concept of mental deficiency as a homogeneous entity characterized simply by slowness of development due to inherited defect was revised. A far flung effect of the reorientation of thinking which followed was to free the normal parents of mentally retarded children from shame and guilt and enable them to bring constructive energies to the solution of the problems of their children. It is not an overstatement to say that this pioneering work in a neglected field was one of the sparks which kindled the present awakening of efforts on behalf of these children.

Perhaps his most significant contribution was made in later studies which identified the child who was without intellectual deficit but who showed characteristics of brain injury in tests, in behavior and in learning. The identification of these children then opened the way toward a more specific and therefore more adequate educational therapy which would take into account their perceptual, conceptual and attention problems. This was the first attempt at a psychologically inclusive systematic description of this new clinical syndrome in child psycho-pathology—the minimally brain-injured child.

Many authorities are of the opinion that the full impact of Dr. Strauss' later work has not yet been felt. His attempt to relate particular kinds of deviant behavior as well as conceptual and perceptual irregularities to organic damage is thought to be a step toward the solution of the problem of the many children who are unresponsive to the usual psychotherapeutic approaches.

The studies in aphasia were interrupted by his death. He had hoped to outline a frame of reference—genetic, pathologic and linguistic—in which this problem could be better understood, the ultimate goal being improved therapeutic methods.

Dr. Strauss' findings and applications have been widely published. He is the author, with Laura E. Lehtinen, of *Psychopathology and Education of the Brain-Injured Child* (Grune & Stratton, New York, 1947), and with Prof. Newell C. Kephart of Purdue University of Volume II of this work, which reports continuing progress in theory and clinic (1955).

Preface

It took us many years to write two books on brain-injured children.* During all the time that these volumes for professional workers were being written and during their reception, we were aware of the need for a book for the parents of these children. Although the professional worker who deals with parents as well as children is equipped to write such a book, we were reluctant to do so. We were always disappointed with books for parents written by professionals because the knowledge was so objective, the experience cross-sectional rather than longitudinal, neither one having been tried in the crucible of the parents' emotions. On the other hand, books written by parents lacked the knowledge and objectivity of the professional. Therefore, we decided to collaborate on a book for parents with a parent of a brain-injured child. In addition, the parent would be a professional writer. Our choice was Mr. Lewis. '

The result of our co-ordinated efforts was the first book of this title.† As the years passed, we believed that the additional experiences and insights we acquired justified a new and more comprehensive book for parents and laymen. We believed also that some of our approaches might be helpful to teachers of both normal and exceptional children, since the brain-injured child sometimes is encountered in regular and special classrooms.

A book for parents of a handicapped child is by its nature not a neutral report on a phenomenon. It must reflect, partly at least, the emotional state in which a parent finds himself when he suffers from his own confusion and doubt in understanding and

---

* Strauss, A. A. and Lehtinen, L. E.: Psychopathology and Education of the Brain-Injured Child, 1947, vol. 1; Strauss, A. A., Kephart, N. C., Lehtinen, L. E., and Goldenberg, S.: Psychopathology and Education of the Brain-Injured Child, New York, Grune & Stratton, 1955, vol. 2.

† Lewis, R. S., Strauss, A. A., and Lehtinen, L. E.: The Other Child, New York, Grune & Stratton, 1951.

rearing such an "otherwise," different being who is still his nearest kin. A book on a handicapped child cannot give detailed prescriptions, like a book on baby care or a book on rearing a normal child. With the normal child in mind, one can nearly describe all the needs and desires and their fulfillment as exhibited by any normal child.

In a handicapped child, the varieties of developmental deviations (even in the small field of brain-injured children) and the varieties of parental reactions are so manifold that this book reflects only the more conspicuous generalities.

Mr. Lewis has attempted to tell our experiences illuminated by the light of his own. This volume, like the earlier one, is not a book which will describe a cure or a definite program for absolute success. It will open the eyes of parents of the "other" child. It is intended to help parents understand the "otherness" of brain-injured children, so that the parents may feel they are not alone.

Through the understanding of the strangeness of an "other" individual, parents may achieve some peace of mind. This is the first step to help.

Alfred A. Strauss, Racine, Wis.
Laura E. Lehtinen, Evanston, Ill.

Postscript

This is the last of the books on the brain-injured child which have come from the pioneering genius of the late Dr. Alfred A. Strauss. The new material in this book, in addition to that contributed by Miss Lehtinen, was dictated to me by Dr. Strauss shortly before his death in the fall of 1957. My role as parent and as one of the writers simply has been to communicate the wisdom of a remarkable physician and psychiatrist, whose contribution to that branch of human understanding called the behavioral sciences has provided an enduring legacy for this and future generations of our children.

Richard S. Lewis, Evanston, Ill.

May, 1960.

The Other
Child

CHAPTER I

An Introduction

No other period in history has produced so much literature about the child as the middle of the twentieth century. His growth and behavior have been charted in minute detail. He has been measured physically, emotionally and intellectually. From these observations, there has evolved a prototypical profile of the child as a developing human organism in the culture of modern America. In the prototype, parents may see the essential image of their child as he moves from one age group to another, achieving levels of performance which characterize normal growth.

Insofar as he follows the charted pattern of development, his growth and much of his behavior are predictable. Within certain age limits, he will walk, talk, ride a bicycle and go to school. Generally, he conforms rather closely to the statistical abstraction which such measurement has created as a definition of normality.

Beyond this, however, there is another child who deviates from the normal profile, whose development appears to be erratic and whose total behavior tends to be nonconforming and unpredictable. We introduce him as the "Other Child." As he grows, he becomes recognizable as otherwise than normal to the degree that his development differs from the normal pattern.

We are concerned in this book with the child who is otherwise than normal as the result of an accident which has damaged the central nervous system, more specifically, the brain. The damage may have occurred before, during or after birth.

To denote the environmental origin of the impairment, we refer to him as brain-injured. In our view, he is a normal child who has acquired a handicap which has caused him to develop and respond to his environment in an other than normal manner.

The brain-injured child we will describe may or may not be physically handicapped. Whether he is or not depends on the location of the brain damage. He is usually the child of normal parents. He appears in every economic, social, national or racial grouping, at every time in history and at every place. He began life in the womb with a normal brain potential. Somewhere along the line of growth, his natural development was disrupted by an accidental event. It may have been a trauma resulting from birth injury, a fall, an automobile accident. Or, the brain tissue may have been damaged by an infection, lack of oxygen or extremely high fever. Or, while the developing child was still in the uterus, the mother may have suffered from an infection, or a disturbance in her own body chemistry which affected the growth of the child.

Whatever the cause, we will not dwell here with how or when the accident happened, but with what has happened and what can be done about it after the fact of brain injury has been established.

In many instances, the presence of brain damage may not be detected early in life if the child is not visibly physically handicapped. He may appear to follow normal patterns of development in many ways; but in many ways he does not. In early childhood, his mental growth may seem ambiguous—sometimes normal, sometimes not. Ambiguities may also appear in his behavior which may seem sometimes normal, sometimes not. It is to the extent that he deviates from the mainstream of normal children that he becomes a problem. And the problem may be more conspicuous in urban surroundings in which conformity in children is stressed than in isolated rural areas.

Brain injury is an accident. It can neither be foreseen nor prepared for. The results are usually drastic, for a fundamental disruption in the life of the victim and his family is produced. Not only is the original potential of the child altered but also the manner and means by which he reaches another potential. One of its conspicuous consequences is anomalous behavior. In discussing behavior, we refer not only to the manner in which the child responds to others but to the totality of his response to his environment.

Another conspicuous consequence of brain injury, one which may not be evident until the child reaches school age, is learning difficulty. It does not necessarily signify a deficiency in intelligence. But, together with deviated behavior, it may prevent him from progressing with his public-school class despite an adequate intellectual potential.

Inevitably, a description of the brain-injured child tends to be comparative. Comparing him with the statistical image of the normal child provides a portrait of his "otherness." He is "otherwise" in relation to his environment and to the manner in which he is expected to perform.

In general, we can portray the Other Child in the ways in which he varies from the normal profile of child development. Physically, he grows like the normal child and his emotional needs are the same. It is in the realm of behavior and learning that he is recognized as "other."

Familial traits which parents expect to see in their children are frequently not visible in him. He does not reflect his environment as adequately as the normal child does. Nor does he cope with it as adequately.

In many instances, the Other Child has special environmental needs. When these are met, as we will show, his behavior deviations tend to decrease and his ability to adjust to normal surroundings improves.

When he reaches school age, the Other Child who shows inability to adjust to or learn in a conventional public school environment may be found to be "retarded" and placed in a class for retarded children if the community provides one. If he cannot be so classified because his intelligence is "normal," he remains a misfit for whom the public school does not provide.

We believe some of his learning and adjustment problems in conventional classes for the retarded are similar to those in the normal classroom. Whether or not the brain-injured child is intellectually retarded, his learning difficulties and adjustment problems are different from those of nonbrain-injured retarded children. The basis of the difference is that brain functioning in the Other Child has been altered by physical destruction of tissue. The brain-injured child is essentially a crippled child even if his crippledness is not visible. While this may appear to be a fine distinction, it is a critical one. Unless it is realized, the mountainous problems this child faces in getting along in ordinary society may not be understood.

Not enough is known about the physiology of the brain to permit the "otherness" of the brain-injured child to be described in physiological terms. If he is not visibly crippled, and in many cases he is not, the effect of brain injury may not be detected by a routine medical examination. It may not be evident on the electroencephalogram. Rather, the effect may show up in the over-all behavior and intellectual peculiarities of the child, tending to become more obvious as he grows older.

As we have indicated, he may or may not be deficient in intelligence. He may merely show behavior difficulties which do not yield to conventional psychotherapeutic methods or learning problems which resist the efforts of teachers and tutors.

Such children who reach school age without being recognized as brain-injured may by then have acquired emotional problems to complicate the picture further. Many of them are found in classes for the mentally handicapped, in special rooms for children with behavior problems or, struggling and misunderstood, in classes for normal children. In many of these the Other Child is frequently unable to make a successful adjustment or adequate academic progress.

Whether or not neuromotor defects are present, the nature of the brain-injured child's handicap is such that placing him in a class of "slow learners" is analogous to putting the physically crippled child on a team of slow runners. The crippled child may be taught to walk and run and the brain-injured child may be taught to learn. But both require teaching programs which take their handicaps into account. In the brain-injured child, the handicap influences the whole range of his activity. The brain is the central station of power and transformation of energy in the human organism. It functions at the signal of the senses which react to stimuli from the outer world.

It is the brain which motivates all effort. It is the architect of the human personality. If it is damaged, it functions irregularly. In consequence, the performance, the personality and the behavior become irregular.

Brain-injured children show disturbances in the brain functions of perception, or the way in which they perceive the world, and in concept formation, or the way in which they think about what they perceive.

In cases where the neuromotor system is not apparently involved in brain damage, there may be no physical sign that brain damage has occurred. The only visible symptom may be the widespread deviation in behavior. And disturbances in perception and thinking may not be suspected as the cause of this deviation. These disturbances show up in the way the child responds to his environment. When they are present, his responses tend to be inadequate compared to the normal expectation, or strange in comparison to the responses of the child who is normal.

Compared to the normal view of reality, the brain-injured child sees his world often as a series of shifting, poorly related scenes in which foreground and background images seem to merge in confusion or in which isolated events, detached from their context are accepted as reality. Yet, all of his sensory organs may be normally acute. Wherein lies the distortion?

It is in the brain that the physical stimuli responded to by the sensory organs may be incorrectly or incompletely selected, sorted and taken in, and erroneously evaluated. Responses to faulty data tend to be wrong responses. And the sum of the child's responses is behavior.

The brain-injured child is not new in human society. Only his identification as such is relatively recent. He is as old as history. He is the child who "fell on his head," the "odd one."

Until rather recently, he was left to his own devices. He went to school as long as he was tolerated there. In a rural region, in which the demands of conformity were not great, he was not particularly conspicuous, especially if his failings could be sheltered by a large family. What became of him at maturity is not known. Many brain-injured children seem to vanish into the general population as they reach maturity.

Because the recognition of the brain-injured child is so recent, we do not know how such children fare as adults. A few years ago, the concept of brain injury as a specific handicap in learning and behavior was shared by only a few researchers.

We know of no reliable index of the number of brain-injured children in the population. Some educators have guessed that five in every thousand children are brain-injured, but there is no reliable statistical evidence to confirm this estimate.

It can be assumed, however, that the number of brain-injured children in the population is increasing with the population. In the last ten years, the difficulties of this child attracted more attention from educators, psychologists and psychiatrists than ever before.

With the rising emphasis on special education for the exceptional child, the brain-injured child has become more conspicuous as the educational problem he represents does not yield to conventional methods of teaching exceptional children. Although we do not know how brain-injured children fare as adults, our observations of those from primary school age to late adolescence indicate that many of them can be educated to lead normal, useful lives.

If we have tended to depict brain injury as a catastrophic event, it is to emphasize the uniqueness of the problem for the child, his parents and the community. The problem contains a big challenge to the resources of all three, but it is a problem that can be dealt with once it is recognized. From this viewpoint, we can suggest a general plan for parents in approaching and dealing with the problem.

One of the critical factors in the approach to it is the attitude of the parents. If it is fatalistic, there is little likelihood of a solution for the child. We regard brain injury as an accident—an unforseeable, unpredictable event which has disrupted the child's natural development. Such an event is no one's fault and blame cannot be assigned to it.

Parents who nurture a feeling of guilt for the child's predicament misdirect the energy they might expend more beneficially in planning for the child's future. While it is futile for parents to dwell on the cause, it is urgently necessary for them to prepare to deal with the result. The Other Child is a particular responsibility. In many instances, it lies within the power of the parents to take positive steps that will enable the child to adjust to normal society.

Medicine, psychotherapy and special education have recognized for years the problems of motor training and emotional adjustment of the brain-injured child who is physically crippled. But those children in whom the results of brain damage appear only in intellectual and behavior areas have not fared so well.

As we have indicated, they are frequently not recognized as brain-injured and hence the nature of their difficulties is not understood. The deviations in their behavior may be confused with the emotional difficulties that appear in the normal child. And emotional disturbances in the brain-injured child tend to mask the basic cause of his deviation.

In many cases, the "misbehavior" of the Other Child may be regarded in the community as willful or as the product of lack of training in the home. And because of such misconstruction, parents frequently find·themselves without community support or sympathy in dealing with the behavior and learning problems the child displays. At the outset, therefore, many parents of brain-injured children find they have to go it alone in seeking a solution to a problem which is often outside their own experience and that of relatives or friends.

Parents have reported they have "run from pillar to post" looking for explanations of the child's enigmatic behavior, only to be told that the child would "straighten out" in time or that he needed more discipline or that he was "emotionally upset."

Well meaning relatives may unwittingly influence postponement of a professional analysis of the child's difficulties by insisting he will "grow out of it." But the brain-injured child may never "grow out of it." His difficulties do not abate with time alone. Instead, they may tend to become more acute unless the proper steps are taken to meet them.

We know of no quick and easy solutions to the behavior and learning difficulties of brain-injured children. These are not dispelled by patent cures or wonder drugs; not yet, at least. And we know of no quick miracles. If there is a miracle, it resides in faith and love—faith that human problems yield to human understanding and love that impels the parents to meet what may appear at the outset to be a formidable challenge.

Awareness that a child is otherwise than normal may come slowly. When it does, the parents' first step is to turn to an expert for a definition of the child's condition. The physician may be able to give a general estimate of the damage. The psychologist may then make a more detailed assessment through observation and tests. The teacher who is especially trained to teach and understand brain-injured children may then take over the job of helping parents educate the child.

The first step in approaching any problem is to determine its nature. In the case of the child who appears otherwise than normal, this requires a diagnosis by experts who include the physician (pediatrician, child neurologist and child psychiatrist), and the psychologist. If the child is found to have been brain-injured, the next step is an evaluation by experts of what his potential may be. To what extent can the child be educated to become reasonably self sufficient and competent as he matures?

Experts may give their opinions, but the parents must make the decisions. If the child is so severely damaged that there is no hope of restituting him by known methods, the decision becomes a choice of keeping him at home or providing for him the protection of an institution.

The borderline beyond which custodial care becomes necessary, we believe, should be defined by the parents in consultation with experts. A great variety of conditions enter into this definition. We cannot state them here. We can suggest only the process by which parents may decide in a rational way.

If the professional prognosis indicates that the child can adjust to normal society, the challenge which the child presents becomes a valid one. Then it is probable that special methods of training and special educational techniques will enable the child to become a competent adult and, of more immediate importance, a reasonably well adjusted child.

If the prognosis indicates the child may not be expected to orient himself to normal society, the area of decision is narrowed to the choice between institutional and home care, provided each has its appropriate training opportunities.

In this book, we are concerned with the child whose prognosis indicates that he can make a reasonable social adjustment with an educational program designed to meet his needs. Mainly, we are concerned with the Other Child in a normal family.

In the broken home or in the home in which the parents' own maladjustment prevents them from dealing effectively with the problem, the situation is much more complex and the effects of the brain injury can no longer be separated from the effects of the inadequate or noxious environment.

We must limit this discussion, too, to the Other Child in the age group after infancy and before pubescence. This is the period when the results of brain injury usually appear and the period when they can be dealt with most effectively.

The dawning awareness that their child is different may involve an intense emotional experience for the parents. Many parents have told us that they reacted initially to the behavior aberrations of the child 'with feelings of humiliation, frustration, inadequacy and despair. In this frame of mind, they could do little to help the child and feared that inadvertently they may have done much to disturb his behavior further by communicating their anxiety to him. It is inevitable that parents should be disturbed when the child is disturbed and that they should feed back to him their disturbance and further increase his. If this cycle is to be broken, the parents must be the ones to break it. What seems to be essential here is a readjustment of many traditional parental attitudes and expectations and this may be achieved by facing the problem, identifying it and planning a program to solve it.

Initially, the parents must become accustomed to the idea that the massive literature about the child rarely describes the brain-injured child. They must prepare to accept the idea that it may be difficult to see the links of identity between him and themselves. Parents tend to identify themselves with their children. With the normal child, this sometimes operates as a means of understanding and fulfilling his needs. Phases of the normal

child's development stir in parents memories of their own childhood. They recall they "did the same thing at his age." Thus,
the continuity of familial characteristics is revealed. In the brain-
injured child, much of this continuity seems to be missing. "Chip
off the old block" characteristics often do not appear to be there,
or if they are present, they appear magnified or distorted. In the
normal child, the parents see an image of themselves reborn into a new life, with a new chance at making the most of it. His
development gives them a vicarious sense of achievement.

But in the brain-injured child, the parental image appears
distorted, the second chance seems to be lost.

Instead of a sense of achievement, the child's inadequate performance may engender feelings of failure and frustration in the
parents. They may regard the child's behavior deviation as the
reflection of some inadequacy in themselves rather than as a
symptom of crippledness in the child. Such feelings inhibit the
parents from acting effectively for the child. They amplify the
confusion not only of the parents but also of the child—to whom
these reactions inevitably are communicated.

Professional help for the child is also help for the parents. It
clears up many of their misgivings and enables them to respond
adequately to the child's needs.

The Other Child does not follow the developmental pattern
his parents expect because he cannot. And he cannot because his
brain functioning has been altered by injury.

The brain-injured child of normal parents differs from his
parents in that they are normal and he, because of accident, is
not. He must be accepted as he is—a disabled human being constantly struggling to cope with his surroundings. However, the
fact that he is "other" should not isolate him from his parents. It
brings him closer to them. He requires understanding and affec-
tion to a greater degree than many normal children, even though
he may not be able to demonstrate this need or return the affec-
tion at an early age. For him, too often, the outer world is a
place of rejection, reproach and confusion. Only his parents
stand between him and its chaos. So, he tends to draw closer to
the family circle for security and reassurance. His frequent misidentification of reality, the scorn or criticism evoked by his in-

appropriate behavior and his poor performance may have made him feel tentative, insecure and withdrawn outside of his home.

The brain-injured child of normal or superior intelligence becomes aware rather early that he is otherwise, sometimes before his parents do. Other children help make him aware of it as they reject or exploit him.

These are some of the secondary consequences of his disability. But, unless the disability is understood, they may not be related by parents and teachers to the primary consequences.

The brain-injured child's disturbances in mental functioning distort his notions of time, space and structure. He may not perceive in the normal way physical structures, like toys or other artefacts, or abstract structures, like games or social organization. When he cannot perceive them adequately, he cannot use or enter into them adequately. He is displaced. The brain-injured child is a natural displaced person, sometimes even in his own home, and the basic job that must be done is to enable him to find his place. Sometimes, we see him at the periphery of a children's game, imitating the activity from the sidelines, but not taking part in it. When the other children shout, he shouts; when they run, he runs. He may shout the wrong words or run the wrong way, but he is playing, too, in imitation. In larger patterns of life experience, his activity may also be peripheral unless he is taught how to perceive these patterns in the normal way so that he can fit into them.

Education for the brain-injured child should start as early as possible. Primary education begins for him at the same age as for the normal child. Delay in his schooling because of his handicap serves only to diminish his learning potential. As we will demonstrate later, a special program of primary education is essential for him. It differs from conventional programs in that it takes into account his specific disability.

In this book, we will discuss the psychopathology, management and education of the brain-injured child. We present a generalized picture of the child. We cannot cover the myriad differences in personality, behavior and intellectual potential in brain-injured children.

While brain-injured children differ individually, all have in common, although to varying degrees, the problem of adjusting to normal society. Can this problem be solved?

It has been our experience that if we devise a program of living and education which takes into account the disabilities of brain injury, we can bring these children more nearly into normal focus, so that their "otherness" becomes indiscernible. In many brain-injured children we can decrease "otherness" so that the child is able to make his way in normal society with considerable independence.

There are, however, some children who do not and cannot respond to any program we know of. They continue to remain, "other."

CHAPTER II

PERCEPTION: Seeing Is Believing

We think of the human brain as the most complex instrument in nature. Modern physiologic research has compared it to a computing machine. Analogue and digital computers have been constructed to perform some of the functions of the human brain more rapidly than the brain can perform them. These machines function in the manner in which the brain is believed to function in a part of its activity. But no machine has yet been devised that even approaches the total performance of the human brain.

The brain is more than a machine. It is an instrumentality for the transformation of energy on a scale so vast that it can be measured only in terms of the totality of human achievement. All of man's structures, from the Pyramids to the Empire State Building, emanate from the brain. The sunburst of the hydrogen bomb, the whirling earth satellites and the countless artefacts of human culture are products of the brain, working through sensory and effector organs and a myriad assortment of tools.

Yet, in comparison with the massive input of electrical energy computing machines require, the brain functions on a minute electrical input, and its discharge of electrical energy is so small that it can be detected only by the most delicate instruments.

Physiologists consider that brain functioning is an electro-chemical process. The mental activities of perception and concept formation are thought of as taking place in an electrical field generated by this process. The operational brain has been imagined by the British physiologist, W. Grey Walter,* as:

A vast aggregation of electrical cells, numerous as the stars of the Galaxy, some ten thousand million of them, through which surge the restless tides of an electrical being relatively thousands of times more potent than the force of gravity. It is when a million or so of these cells repeatedly fire together that the rhythm of their discharges becomes measurable in frequency and amplitude.

In its bony, cranial housing, the brain is shielded from the outer world. It has no direct contact with the external environment of the organism. It corresponds with the environment through data fed to it by the sensory organs and acts on the outer world through the effector organs of the neuromotor system. Data reported by the sensory organs are registered in and "recognized" by the brain in a process called perception, integrated into patterns of thinking by a process called concept formation and stored for future use in the cellular vaults of the living memory.

From the time radiant energy, sound vibrations and chemical stimuli begin to bombard the sensory organs of the infant, the brain is constantly responding to the outer world. In its responses, it shapes the activity of the organism into well defined patterns. These response patterns are called behavior. One would expect that the responses of individuals to the same environmental stimuli would be similar and that consequently their general behavior would be similar. Mass measurement of the child indicates that this is so.

But let us suppose that one of the mental processes governing the organism's response to its environment is not functioning in the normal manner. In that case, the behavior of the organism would tend to vary from the normal pattern. From this viewpoint, we can examine some of the behavior aberrations of the brain-injured child and explain in general terms some of his difficulties.

Injury to the brain, if severe enough, alters the function of this organ over the whole range of its activity. It may result in paralysis, convulsions, blindness, deafness, loss of speech or in other defects of the nervous system. But whether or not these

° W. Grey Walter: "The Living Brain."

gross manifestations of brain damage are present, a more subtle disruption in brain functioning may have been caused by injury. The functions of perception and concept formation may have been altered. And the alteration may not be detectable except through the behavior of the child. The child who has suffered such a disability may not display it until he has reached the age of two, three, or four, when he is expected to conform to commonly accepted patterns of behavior. The deviation at first may appear small. But as he grows older, it enlarges and parents ask themselves: What is wrong?

The perceptually disabled child does not receive and evaluate the messages of his sensory organs in the normal way, even though these organs may be unimpaired. Consequently, his responses to stimuli tend to be other than normal and his behavior appears "otherwise." In the brain-injured child, we may trace some behavior anomalies to a physiologic source—a damaged organ.

It has been our experience that certain types of aberrated behavior and learning difficulties are the results of brain damage. This does not mean that all behavior deviations or all learning difficulties can be attributed to brain damage. Much of the behavior difficulty of the brain-injured child, as well as of the normal child, may be a result of emotional disturbance. The services of an expert are essential in finding the basis of these difficulties.

In the brain-injured child, we can relate much of the inadequacy of response this child demonstrates to the malfunctioning of the perceptual process. It may be helpful for parents to consider what this process is.

Let us think of perception generally as an activity of the brain between sensation and thought—as the method by which the outer world is "seen" by the brain.

The eye records gradations of light, but the images seen take form in the brain and central nervous system. Similarly, the organs of hearing, touch, taste and smell detect various combinations of matter and energy within their range. But the perception of these stimuli is, again, a neuropsychic or neuromental process.

The process known as kinesthetic perception records the position and tension of the muscles in relation to the total musculature. It also records the position of the body in relation to the earth's center of gravity through the balance mechanism in the inner ear. Perception, then, is the process by which stimuli affecting sensory organs are organized into structures or patterns abstracted from the outer world. The manipulation of these abstracts into modes of thinking once they have been impressed on the brain is the process of concept formation, or conception.

Man has sought to extend the range of his sensory organs or to correct their malfunctioning by mechanical means. Glasses and hearing aids correct the operation of the organs, and telescopes, microscopes, sound-ranging detectors and radar extend the range. But these devices are meaningless unless what they detect can be adequately perceived by the brain.

Research in psychology has shown that the perceptual process is basically the same in all normal human beings. It is not certain whether, physiologically, ways of perceiving the world are inherent or whether much of perception is learned. It can be said, however, that whether the process is inherent or learned, the course of development it takes from infant to adult is universally comparable.

One of the characteristics of perception is that it occurs as a whole—all at once, nothing first. A photograph of someone we know is recognized at first glance without an examination of details. A musical phrase is identified in its entirety, not note by note. In normal perception, the whole is recognized at once, along with all of its significant parts. We see the total figure before we examine the details. We see the whole first. It is when the whole is not instantly recognizable that we break it down to search for clues in its components. From this view of perception, the perceptual difficulties of the brain-injured child become evident. Frequently, he does not perceive the whole. Instead, he sees one of the parts as a lesser whole. The result is distortion.

In normal perception, the whole is arranged in terms of figure and background. We do not give equal value to the myriad sensory reports that may be involved in a single percept. The foreground figure and the background are clearly resolved. Their relationship is obvious and consistent. When we look at a photograph of someone we know, we recognize the person irrespective of what clothes he happens to be wearing. When we hear a known musical phrase, we recognize it irrespective of the instrument producing the sound or the impromptu variations of the player. Thus, a known figure can be identified regardless of shifts in its background. Cousin George, photographed in front of the Taj Mahal, is still Cousin George. "The Star Spangled Banner" is recognized whether it is played by bagpipes or a military band.

Most of the activities and situations we perceive take place against a background of varying visual, auditory, tactual or kinesthetic stimuli. Normally, we are able to sort out substance from shadow, figure from ground without conscious effort. But the brain-injured child with a perceptual disturbance frequently cannot do this. He is not able all the time to see the same whole with the same figure-ground relationship as the normal person does. Instead, the brain-injured child tends to be transfixed by one of the parts, which leaps into his foreground as a smaller whole and reduces the normally perceived whole to background status. Consequently, the perceptually disturbed child may not receive the same image as the normal child does from the same set of stimuli. This is the basis for much of the brain-injured child's misconstruction of reality, a factor of enormous consequence in shaping his total behavior.

Because of his inability to organize stimuli in the normal way, the brain-injured child is apt to respond to a detail in a scene or situation rather than to the entirety. Normal persons may do so, too, but as a matter of choice. That is, the normal individual may prefer to react to the detail rather than to the whole; but in order for the preference to exist he must perceive both. The perceptually handicapped person has no choice. He perceives the whole only in terms of the detail and it is the detail which dictates his response.

Such a disability results in an endless sequence of perceptual errors or "misconceptions" of reality. At the seashore, a perceptually handicapped child with excellent vision sighted a sail far out. He wanted to know what was sticking out of the water. A sailboat, he was told. Later, when the entire sailboat appeared on a billowing crest, he asked, again, what it was. A sailboat, he was told again, impatiently. "But a sailboat sticks up," he said, puzzled.

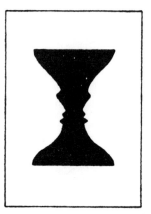

Fig. 1.—Ambiguous figure after Rubin. A vase or two faces. The normal person will see the ambiguity. The brain-injured person may vacillate or see only one pattern.

Can we determine how the brain-injured child's perceptual handicap alters his view of the world from that of the normal child? To some extent, this can be done by psychological tests. It may be illustrated by the response of a brain-injured child to the following sequence:

For example, what does this drawing represent? Two rectangles. It seems to.

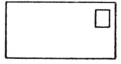

And here we have a V.

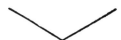

And here, a trough, or an exaggerated letter M.

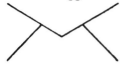

And here, two signal flags.

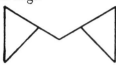

Ah, but here is an envelope.

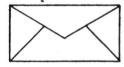

Back where we started—the two rectangles become an envelope with a stamp on it.

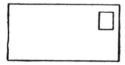

The normal person sees the progression:

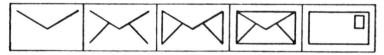

The brain-injured may see this:

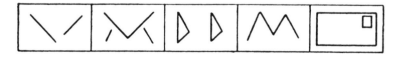

Would he be led to perceive the rectangles as an envelope? Perhaps not. Does this mean he is less intelligent? No, it indicates he is not perceiving what the normal person perceives.

The "V" he might perceive as two lines; the trough as a "V" and two lines; the two flags as disembodied triangles or two kites; the back of the envelope as the letter "M," and the front of the envelope as two rectangles or a house with a window in it.

Such misidentification may be made in the auditory, tactual and kinesthetic sensory fields as well as in vision.

We might summarize the perceptual difficulties of the brain-injured child by saying that he fails to see "the point" or that he does not get "the picture." This deficiency applies to social as well as physical situations.

In a game of softball, the perceptually handicapped child may experience a series of difficulties. First, he may not be able to hit the ball with a bat because this involves a high degree of co-ordination between perceptual and motor functions. He may not be able to tell where the ball is in relation to himself or the bat. But after constant practice, he can be trained to hit the ball. When he does so, a variety of stimuli are set up. One or more of the opposing players chase the ball, and other members of the team in the field shift position. While the batter may "know" he is supposed to run to first base, a detail of the scene, such as a fielder running after the ball, may swerve him from the objective of reaching first base and the batter, too, may start to run after the ball.

Children tend to be quite sophisticated about automobiles, air-planes, even military rockets. They can distinguish between makes, models and types, a feat involving the perception of form through contour and detail. Brain-injured children may also discern these distinctions part of the time, but not all of the time. What is the difference? In his identification of the make and model of an automobile, for example, the perceptually handicapped child may pin his faith on a detail, such as the rear fins or the grille. Such a detail may or may not be characteristic of the whole.

Adequate perception of form depends on the ability to perceive the whole and the relationships of its parts to each other and to the whole. Where perception of the whole is lacking, the relationships are lost. Thus, all autos with twin tail pipes may seem to be the same make and model to the perceptually handicapped child.

Identification of structures requires an overlay of learning and experience, which is summarized, in the identifying process, by naming. Once we name a thing, we have incorporated its structure in our minds. The name symbolizes the essential differences and similarities which make the object unique.

Usually, the name of a thing conjures up its total structure and the experiences we have had with it. Naming is also a conceptual activity in which the name refers to a class of objects with over-all similarities but individual differences. The term, "building," for example, refers to a class of structures containing many different types. Abstractly, the term, "building," may be considered a whole in the area of concept formation, and various types of buildings as its parts. There is evidence that the brain-injured child carries over his inability to perceive the whole to the area of concept formation. That is, he may fail to distinguish between a class of objects and a single object as part of the class. To him, a building may invariably be a house and he may not see the relatedness of a school, a church or the state capitol as "buildings"; their relationship may be clearer if they are referred to as schoolhouse, House of God or state house.

Little J. was once told that a culvert was a "kind of bridge." For many years, the percept of the culvert confused him whenever he saw what was described to him as a bridge. How could the Chain of Rocks Bridge at St. Louis be a bridge when it was so much bigger than a culvert?

In normal perception, the individual does not lose sight of the totality while examining its details. He is able to keep both in mind at the same time. As he examines each detail, he "holds" it in relation to other details and to the whole. But perceptually disturbed persons do not seem to be able to "hold" these relationships successfully, especially when confronted with complex structures. Even though they may be shown how to perceive the whole, they may tend to lose it when shifting to one of the parts.

The brain-injured child may be able to perceive a figure, such as a square. When asked to draw it, he must shift to its parts. In drawing the square, he is likely to leave its corners unconnected. He has drawn a series of lines which have a spatial relationship but which do not complete the figure of a square. Sometimes, the perceptually handicapped child may not perceive a square as a structural unity of four lines; he may see only four lines. He may draw the lines, but he does not draw the square.

Mathematically, we say that the whole is the sum of its parts. Is it? In perception, the whole is frequently much more than the sum of its parts. The brain-injured child may perceive all of the parts, but he may not perceive the whole. And the importance of seeing the whole is paramount in the perceptual process, since normal responses usually are made to wholes, rather than parts.

Let us apply this distinction to the classroom where the brain-injured child is having a hard time. He is coloring with the other children. He may be able to color up to a single line, but he cannot color within the confines of a square as the others can. Why not? As we have indicated, he may not perceive the square as a unified figure, but only as a series of lines—and which side of the lines should he color up to?

Suppose one child exhibits this failing in a kindergarten. What can the teacher do to help him? If the child's perceptual difficulty is understood, the remedy is not mysterious. For one such child, a cardboard mask was made with a square area cut out in the center. The child was shown how to lay the mask down on the paper and move the crayon about within the confines of the cut-out until it came in contact with all four sides. In this way, the child produced a colored square patch, instantly visible against the white paper when the cardboard was removed. After some practice with the mask, the child looked at his work and said: "It sticks out, it sticks out." For the first time, this child of eight had seen clearly the differentiation of a figure from its background. He had learned to perceive the figure of a square.

In normal perception, there is often ambiguity between foreground and background or figure and background, especially where the background is patterned. But in spite of the patterning of background, the person with normal perceptual ability can isolate the figure once he has "seen" it or differentiated it from the background.

The brain-injured child frequently cannot isolate the figure against a patterned background. Even if he has been shown the figure, he may not be able to hold it against the interference of the background patterns. This perceptual instability appears in hearing as well as in vision. Its recognition is of considerable importance in determining the brain-injured child's educational program and teaching environment.

It is apparent that if the child's focus oscillates between figure and ground in the perception of visual and auditory stimuli, so would it shift in the perception of situations requiring certain modes of conduct, such as games, the classroom or the entertainment of visitors in the home.

In the classroom, this oscillation of focus, or attention, shows up as distractibility. As we will see in a later chapter, the brain-injured child in the primary grades requires a special kind of classroom to control this oscillation, especially at the outset of his learning experience.

Perceptual malfunctioning affects the child's responses to all sensory data over the entire range of his receptivity. Thus, it sharply reduces his ability to "structure" or organize environmental stimuli into normal physical and social patterns. In using the term, "structure," we refer to the organization of parts in the whole, whether it is a physical structure, like a school building, or a social structure, like the Cub Scouts.

The term, "structure," then, denotes the organization of a series of percepts, or experiences, into a pattern, whether it relates to physical or social environment, or is tangible or intangible.

The architect structures a building when he draws the blueprints. The scientist seeks to organize nature into structures of natural law. The schoolman structures education into programs of teaching. The race track bettor's "system" is a structure. So are batting averages, assembly lines, insurance actuarial tables, vacation itineraries, weddings and wakes.

Human activity in modern society is structured for the individual from the day of birth. The child who fails to perceive adequately the physical and social structures of his environment begins life under a formidable handicap. This is the essential dilemma for the brain-injured child. Not only may his initial structuring of his environment be inadequate from the normal viewpoint, but also his ability to structure at more sophisticated levels as he matures. Thus, perceptual errors early in life are perpetuated. Distortions of reality persist even as the child grows in experience. Even when the child's perceptual ability has improved through maturation and special education he is delivered only with great difficulty from the bonds of his earlier misshapen structurings.

We have discussed perception as an instantaneous decoding of sensory message, but we must also consider its ultradimensional characteristic of time. The temporal aspect of perception involves the continual modification of percepts by new stimuli being integrated with the old.

In the perception of new stimuli, there is the instantaneous amalgamation of the new with the memory-stored impressions of the past, so that the older structure is altered. At the same time, the older structure is evoked to modulate the new impression. In this way, perception takes place both in space and time. Existing percepts are constantly being "modernized" or "updated" in terms of this amalgamation.

We refer to existing structures to which we relate new phenomena as "experience" and we tend to evaluate new impressions in the light of experience. Thus, the temporal aspect of perception tends to influence behavior insofar as we respond to the new in terms of the old.

The gulf between one generation and the other exists at the perceptual as well as at the conceptual level of mental activity. The adult may respond differently than the child to the same set of stimuli. In terms of experience, the adult tends to perceive stimuli differently than does the child. For junior, a puppy appears to be a marvelous plaything; for mother, it is an added responsibility.

In normal development, the acquisition of life experience tends to alter behavior. Human responses are not the same in maturity as in childhood or adolescence, although there may be general similarities. Patterns of response undergo continual change as percepts are altered by the continuous inflow of stimuli. In the process of perception, then, there is a continuity of organization which affects and is affected by the impact of new stimuli. The erroneous impressions received by the brain-injured child tend to make for faulty perception of new stimuli, so that the child's ability to perceive more complex structures is handicapped.

The child's primary confusion in foreground-background configurations extends from visual and auditory images to abstract social structures and modes of conduct dictated by them. His faulty structurings affect his perception of new stimuli and are affected by the addition of the new misconstruction. Thus, his perceptual deviation tends to be perpetuated and his responses, or behavior, tend to continue out of alignment with the normal pattern.

The physiologic condition for learning may be considered as a continuity of structuring which allows the existing structure to be reformed by new experience. But if the existing structure is faulty, and the new experience is faultily perceived, the faultiness is perpetuated in the modified structure.

This condition has an important bearing on the education of the brain-injured child. Educators generally consider that by the age of six the normal child has acquired sufficient experience to promote his readiness for formal education. That is, he has developed sufficient perceptual ability in distinguishing forms and relating them in space to learn how to read and count.

In the brain-injured child, this "readiness" may not be apparent. The experiences of drawing, coloring and the matching of shapes in puzzles and games which promote perceptual readiness in the normal child do not necessarily promote such readiness in the Other Child.

The perceptual difficulties of the brain-injured child have blocked his readiness. Therefore, he is not ready for school at the same age as the normal child. Does this mean he might become "ready" at a later age—at eight instead of six? Some school administrators take this view. But it has been our experience that the brain-injured child does not become "ready" by time alone.

Instead, he has to be helped to become ready. This means that the perceptual skill which the normal child acquires through experience with games and puzzles must be taught to the brain-injured child. This child must be taught how to perceive so that he can learn, and he should be taught as early as possible. Unless this is done, he cannot learn adequately, if at all, in a primary school environment.

We have discussed in general terms why this is so. The experiences he may have shared with normal children have not promoted reading or number readiness in him, as in them, because he has failed to perceive these experiences adequately. And unless these misperceptions are corrected at an early age, he may not develop the ability to perceive what is being taught later. Moreover, his foreground-background confusion makes it difficult for him to focus on the teaching material. In the classroom itself, whisperings or outside noises have the same power to capture his attention as the lesson. He tends to be distracted from the situational focus by the intrusion of background or peripheral stimuli.

Such distractibility displayed by the brain-injured child might be dismissed as "limited span of attention."

The phrase is semantically dubious. A child who does not pay attention to the lesson is obviously attending to something else. If the classroom situation is loosely structured, to him, extraneous sights and sounds leap into his foreground and he shifts his focus to them.

Inattention in the normal child is usually voluntary; in the brain-injured child, involuntary. The normal child may decide that the men outside trimming trees are much more interesting than the lesson, but while he is watching them he is also conscious of the lesson and can swing back to it. When the brain-injured child is distracted, his shift in focus is not a conscious choice. He loses awareness of the lesson, or it becomes an insignificant background detail, and the distraction becomes the whole show.

It is necessary to structure the classroom for the brain-injured child so that he can clearly perceive its focus and hold it against distractions. This is done by eliminating as many distractions as possible so that the child learns by experience what the focus is. When the classroom is so structured for him, his "span of attention" seems magically to "grow," that is, his ability to perceive the classroom in the normal way has grown. His perceptual field has been organized so that he can function as a pupil instead of as a distraught child.

Learning proceeds from the organization of the child's perceptual field. We have seen that the perceptual process is temporal insofar as past and present sensory data interact, so that what is being perceived today affects and is affected by what has been perceived yesterday. It is therefore reasonable to expect that the earlier the brain-injured child receives training in perceptual organization, the firmer becomes his ability to draw on the time line of experience. As this ability increases, the deviation of his responses in learning and behavior decreases. Conversely, the longer his education is put off, the more difficult it becomes to teach him and the more he is cheated of normal learning experience.

That is why we say that the educable brain-injured child should start school at the age the normal child does, whether "ready" or not. If he is not "ready," then he has to be helped to become so. He does not become "ready" by idling at home.

The earlier the brain-injured child is taught how to perceive as normally as possible, the more adequate become his responses. Most of us are aware that the reiteration of stimuli modifies percepts. Sometimes we seek repetition in order to "get the picture." Reiteration enables the normal person to revise impressions if they are at first erroneous. But the perceptually handicapped child cannot make the correction if he does not perceive the error.

Consider the person who is buying a house for the first time. After his initial tour, he may find he has only a vague impression of what he has seen. It did have a large kitchen, but what of the dining room? Was there a dining room? The interested buyer looks at the house again and again, until he has a firm idea of the total structure and the relationship of its parts. Even then, the house continues to "change" after he moves in as new relationships appear.

Unless the brain-injured child is taught to perceive properly, reiteration, such as that practiced in classes for retarded children, may not enable him to correct error but may, instead, entrench the error.

Perception is a developmental process, in which older forms undergo continual modification as new relationships appear. For the normal person, the process is continuous. In the brain-injured individual, it may be discontinuous insofar as new relationships may be inadequately perceived and fail to modify existing structures.

The perceptual confusion of the brain-injured child may be compared with that of the normal person confronted by new experience or stimuli he cannot relate to any previous experience.

One of the functions of military training is to enable the soldier to perceive the structure of combat situations to which he might be exposed. Inexperienced troops who cannot perceive the nature of an action become confused and cannot perform the minimal functions required for survival. But veterans do not become confused and can perform. They have had experience in structuring these situations. Thus, "green" troops exhibit one form of behavior under fire while experienced troops exhibit another.

Normal persons frequently misidentify the nature of unfamiliar phenomena which does not relate to past experience. During World War II in the European Theater, replacements tended to mistake the rumble of heavy artillery shells passing overhead for a convoy of trucks on the road. When the first jet fighters appeared over Britain, they were mistaken for bombs. The early V-1 flying bombs were confused with jet aircraft. And the first bombings by supersonic V-2 rockets were thought to be gas main explosions.

One of the most widely publicized perceptual anomalies of the post-war years has been the advent of the "flying saucers." Of 5,500 reported sightings investigated by the U. S. Air Force between 1947 and 1958, all but 2 per cent have been explained as weather balloons, reflections of searchlights on clouds, conventional aircraft, meteorites, sun dogs, fixed stars or birds. Yet, out of these perceptual experiences, there has come in the last decade a popular image of the flying saucer, even though objective evidence has failed to confirm the existence of such an outré vehicle.

At best, human perception tends to be precarious, often ambiguous and never final. It is constantly undergoing alteration by new experience and continually must be evaluated in terms of past experience. In this light, the perceptual difficulties of the brain-injured child might be faintly imagined.

We say that seeing is believing or, "I'm from Missouri—Show me." Not seeing, but perceiving, is believing, and even then we cannot always be sure of what we see.

For what we see, hear, taste, touch or smell acquires meaning in terms of frames of reference. What happens in the perceptual process when basic frames of reference are distorted or unavailable? For example, how would a man perceive his environment in a condition of "weightlessness" or "free fall" when the organism is no longer oriented by gravity? When man is no longer "attached" by the umbilicus of gravity to the center of the earth, which way is "up" or "down"? Many persons are familiar with the feeling of disorganization when an airplane banks in a sharp turn and centrifugal force momentarily supplants the force of gravity. The whole universe seems to tilt. The earth is beside us, instead of underneath us. Then we shift back to the conventional frame of reference as the turn is completed and the airplane levels out, so that we are once more perpendicular to the center of the earth's gravity. Man's ability to perceive his environment adequately outside of his conventional geophysical frame of reference has been an important research subject in space medicine. Unquestionably, the spacemen of the near future will have to be trained to perceive in the environment of space before they can function in it.

Man has proven himself to be perceptually adaptable. He can function in more than one frame of reference, in several different kinds of environment. The same individual can learn to function at maximum efficiency for survival at the South Pole or at the intersection of State and Madison Streets in Chicago, where survival probably requires greater perceptual ability than it does at the South Pole.

We consider perception as a serial process, involving a complex system of integration between sense fields and past and present sensory impressions. In the beginning, certain basic reactions occur spontaneously in the organism as the result of its biologic growth. These basic reactions, however, become a minor part of the perceptual process as it becomes more sophisticated with experience. By far the greater part of our perceptual function results from the elaboration and modification of these basic reactions by experience and learning.

Consequently, when we talk about an individual's perceptual ability, we must relate it to the individual's stage of development. One cannot compare the percepts of two individuals without considering their relative developmental states, for the percepts of the individual with greater experience are bound to differ qualitatively from those of the individual with lesser experience.

We alluded earlier to the gulf between generations, in which the oldster views the world differently than the youngster. The perception of the child is different from that of the adult. It is so different that adult perception cannot be considered simply as a modification of childhood perception. Colloquially, this distinction is recognized in the rather ordinary sayings: "He's not the man he was at 30," or "She's not the same child she used to be." Perceptually speaking, these statements are more literal than figurative. The man of 60 is not the same man he was at 30. His physiology has changed. So have his percepts and other mental processes. He has the same identity, but his behavior, outlook and physical structure have altered.

It appears evident, then, that the effect of any disturbance of the perceptual process on the individual will vary with the individual's stage of development at the time the disturbance occurs. A congenital perceptual disturbance, that is, one which is present when the child is born, presents different problems than one which occurs at later stages in life.

We have seen that perceptual disturbance, arising from brain injury, can occur before, during or after birth, that is, at any time in the life of the individual. It may occur in old age and frequently does as the result of a stroke. It follows that the child with a perceptual disability at the time of birth would require more intensive training in perception than the individual whose perceptual structures were normal before he acquired the handicap.

In the process of perception, the individual relates himself to an environmental scheme. The critical aspect of perception is the relationships which are perceived. If the relationships are faultily perceived, the individual's success in relating himself to his environment suffers. The faultiness tends to be perpetuated through the temporal sequences of percept building, unless it is corrected by special education.

The essential nature of perception, as a sensory-mental function, is the organization of relationships. We perceive relatively, not absolutely. We are aware of heat and cold in relation to the normal body temperature of 98.6 degrees Fahrenheit. We know when morning comes on a cloudy day because it is lighter than the night; we do not need to have blinding sunlight tell us a new day has arrived.

It is from the awareness of relationships that learning springs and intellectual activity proceeds. But the appreciation of relationships involves more than the mere registration of sensory data; it involves "output" as well as "input." That is, the perception of new stimuli is affected by the existence of a related perceptual structure just as this mental structure is affected by the new sensory data.

Thus, we think of perception as two-way communication between organism and its environment, in which the external stimuli modify and are modified by the internal structure. The newborn infant hears a shrill sound, but his mother hears a train whistle and grandpa hears the eight o'clock express. The percepts of a number of persons receiving an identical stimulus may differ quite remarkably.

On the Saturday evening before Easter Sunday, 1947, the inhabitants of Coatesville, Indiana, heard a rushing roar which some of them thought was Pennsylvania Railroad's Jeffersonian from St. Louis arriving a bit ahead of schedule. They were wrong. It was a tornado which wrecked one third of the community. For some time after that experience, Coatesville residents experienced a pang of apprehension when they heard the Jeffersonian highballing toward the town until reassured by its whistle.

As awareness of relationships expands, knowledge grows and the individual is able to respond more adequately to situations or events. When relationships are perceived in a faulty manner, they may add to an already imperfect structure. It is the adequacy of the perception of new experiences, not the experiences in themselves, which promotes adequacy of response.

We think of perception as a process in which the thing registering on the sensory organs modifies and is modified by related, preexisting mental structures. The two-way process involves input, or the activation of the sensory organ by a stimulus, and output, or the modification (interpretation) of the stimulus in the brain.

It is our belief that the faultiness of perception in brain-injured children resides in the total perceptual process, not in any "part of it" if, indeed, the process can be broken down into "parts." Some investigators tend to think of perceptual disturbance as a distortion of input, like so-called "mirror vision" where the individual sees things upside down. From this viewpoint, one would be tempted to conclude that if only the sensory image can be corrected, the perceptual disturbance will be eliminated.

Obviously, a defect in the sensory organ would interfere with the perceptual process. But to consider, for example, only the adequacy of the visual image on the retina of the eye, is like assuming a radio will play because it is tuned to a signal. Whether or not it plays, of course, depends on what is done with the signal in the radio's electronic components. And whether or not an individual perceives a stimulus depends on what is done with the signal in the infinitely more complex "circuits" of the central nervous system. In vision, the functioning of the perceptual process depends not only on the adequacy of the retinal image, but on what is done with the image.

Although we tend to describe perception as a sequence of physiologic activities, we do not believe the process can be broken down into components of activity. Rather, it must be considered as a unified design. In the organism, there is no demarcation between the stages of the perceptual process and there should be none in our thinking about it.

A disturbance in perception may occur anywhere in the process. It may be a disturbance of the sense organs, of the integrative mechanisms in the central nervous system or in the response of the organism modifying the signal. Wherever the disturbance occurs, it interferes with and distorts the picture which the child builds up of the world around him and consequently affects his behavior. The existence of a perceptual disturbance, therefore, does not necessarily mean that one or more sensory organs are impaired.

When we consider perception as a two-way proposition, we can better appreciate the interaction between the organism and its environment. Each affects and modifies the other unceasingly. Consider, for example, the automatic elevator in which some of the characteristics of the human nervous system are imitated electrically. One presses the button. The elevator "perceives" the signal, including the floor of its origin, and "responds" by arriving at the floor and opening its doors. The elevator then moves to the next floor in its signal sequence. Involved modifications of the elevator's behavior can be built into it. One of these is especially ingenious. It might be called a "reassurance" response.

In the older types of automatic elevators, one simply pressed the button and waited for the lift to arrive. The person signalling the elevator had no way of knowing whether the signal had been received unless he could hear the elevator start or until it actually arrived. As a consequence of the lack of immediate perceptible response by the elevator, there was a tendency by signallers to keep on pushing the button until a response could be perceived. This caused excess wear on the delicate contact points of the signalling mechanism.

Some newer elevator systems are equipped with a signalling device which lights up as soon as it is activated. In this way, the elevator responds to the signaller with its own signal. It signals back a message, saying, in effect, "okay, I'm coming." Such a message reassures the signaller. More significantly, it seems to modify his behavior insofar as it persuades him it is not necessary to keep on pressing the button.

One might consider the analogy of the automatic elevator to the human nervous system rather crude, but the fact remains that automatic elevator circuits are displacing human operators in office and apartment buildings and hotels all over the country.

Automation provides a dramatic analogy to the human nervous system which can hardly be denied, insofar as automatic machinery displaces human beings in many industrial, commercial and service occupations. What is even more dramatic in the analogy is the fact that a disturbance in the "perceptual mechanism" of an automatic machine disrupts its functioning and alters its behavior—as in the human organism.

When this occurs to a machine, the operator does not punish the machine or abandon it. He sends for a repairman. And one does not punish or abandon the brain-injured child for behavior difficulties arising out of a perceptual abnormality. One determines what can be done to help the child function more normally. We cannot "repair" the brain-injured child, but we can teach him how to modify his behavior aberrations.

Perceptual disability is one of the brain-injured child's invisible handicaps. It often is not the only one. He may also be handicapped in the manipulation of ideas abstracted from the outer world. He may be disabled in the "higher" process of conception, or thinking.

CHAPTER III

CONCEPTION: Believing Is Behaving

We have discussed perception as the process by which impressions of the outer world are received and organized in the brain. Beyond perception appears a further organizing process by which impressions are shaped and reshaped into formulas for decision and action. This process is called conception, or concept formation.

While we speak of perception and conception as though each were a separate activity, modern psychological research regards these processes as aspects of unified mental functioning. From this viewpoint, a child who has suffered a perceptual disability is likely also to show disturbances in conception, or abstract thinking, at least insofar as his thinking reflects his perceptual distortion.

Since conception plays a major role in programming human activity, it would appear that much of the brain-injured child's "otherness" is a behavioral symptom of his conceptual difficulties. His responses at the perceptual level may be faulty and his notion of how he ought to behave, at the conceptual level, may be confused or erroneous.

Recognition of perceptual-conceptual malfunctioning in the brain-injured child provides an approach to programs of special education and behavior reorientation for him. The approach takes into account the child's difficulties at both levels of mental activity. On this foundation, methods that will help the child overcome these difficulties can be devised when the nature of the difficulties is generally understood.

In order to clarify the nature of these difficulties in conception, it is essential to get a clear picture of the conceptual process.

The interaction of perception and conception is commonly recognized in the English language by the substitution of phrases relating to the perceptual process for phrases relating to concept. We say, "I see," when we mean, "I understand." We have just used the phrase, "to get a clear picture," when we mean "have a clear understanding" in discussing a mental process which, of course, cannot be "seen" or "pictured" in a visual-perceptual sense. If we cannot see "the picture" or the idea perceptually, how do we "see" it? And what do we "see"? Presumably, what we "see" is a new and more complex relationship in the percepts which have been abstracted (taken) from the outer world in the perceptual process.

In conception, the brain works over these percepts or abstracts, organizing and reorganizing them, tier upon tier, so to speak, into increasingly complex structures. Conception may be said to differ from perception in that it can take place without immediate sensory activity.

Perception is activated by stimuli from the outer world, but thinking on the conceptual level may occur with or without immediate stimuli. In conception, we manipulate the abstracts we have already acquired through perception and when a relationship suddenly emerges in abstract thinking, we "see" a pattern which was not "visible" to us, or which did not occur to us, before. In total mental functioning, perception and conception involve input and output processes, wherein the outer world acts on the brain, and the brain acts on the outer world.

Residents of a river bottoms community perceive that with prolonged spring rains and melting snow, the river is rising. Past experience has shown them that when these conditions occurred their homes and businesses were flooded. They give the situation some thought in the light of previous experience. They decide to build a levee to contain the river. Thus, at the conceptual level, a program is made by which the residents act on their environment.

The adequacy of abstract thinking is largely dependent on the adequacy of the data which have been abstracted in perception from the real world. Thus, the thinking of the brain-injured child is affected by faulty perception and misconstruction of reality. In addition, however, the brain-injured child's difficulty in perceiving figure-ground organization may also interfere at the conceptual level with the structuring of perceptual experience.

Concept formation requires enough experience so that data, from which concepts can be built, are available. It also requires the ability to organize the data into a scheme which will enable the individual to act effectively and realistically in relation to his environment.

The brain-injured child may have a sufficient quantity of experience, but he may not have been able to abstract sufficient data from it. He has trouble developing concepts for the further reason that his experiences are not well integrated and he cannot manipulate them freely. Thus, the experiences which promote learning readiness for the normal child do not necessarily promote this readiness to the same degree in the Other Child. The Other Child must then be made ready by a teaching program which enables him to organize his experiences more adequately.

One of the most important aspects of conception in which the brain-injured child is frequently deficient is the ability to generalize. Generalization requires the ability to discern similarities in objects, situations or experiences which may be dissimilar in many respects.

The detection of the similarities in different things is a way of relating these things to each other, or of tying them together. The individual who cannot detect these similarities cannot generalize from things, situations and experiences and thus cannot organize them for future reference.

One of the reasons some brain-injured children appear to have unusually good memories may be related to the inability to generalize, and thus "lose" particulars in the larger framework of a generalization. The Other Child may tend to recall a particular detail long after the normal person has merged it into the larger pattern of generalization and forgotten it. Generalizing is a conceptual way of "seeing" the whole from a group or series of parts which may have striking dissimilarities, but important or fundamental similarities.

It will be recalled that J., who was told that a culvert was "a kind of bridge," could not understand that a two mile structure spanning the Mississippi River was also a bridge. How could two things so dissimilar have the same name? He could not grasp the idea that the word, "bridge," could refer to one structure and at the same time refer to a whole class of structures of different sizes and shapes but which had one characteristic in common— they spanned something.

J. also had difficulty in mobilizing his experiences with water. Water ran in the tub, in Fall Creek, in White River and in Niagara Falls. He could not decide whether this meant that there were different kinds of water, such as a bathtub kind, a creek kind or a river kind, or whether water might exist in a variety of locations. Being unable to generalize about watercourses and water, he would attempt to relate percepts of new bodies of water to the water he had already perceived by asking: "Will it wet me? Do fish swim in it? Can I sail a boat on it?"

Eventually, J. mastered the concept of water and the fact that it could be called a river, a creek, a run, a stream, etc. and still be water no longer puzzled him, but his tendency to think in terms of particular kinds persisted. One day, he saw Lake Michigan and was told it was a large body of water. "Is it the deep kind?" he asked.

The brain-injured child's difficulty in generalization is, again, relating parts into wholes. He may be confused when an object he is familiar with is grouped with similar objects and the grouping has a name different from that of the familiar object. A child watched workmen laying brick in a wall. He picked up a piece of brick and brought it into the kitchen.

"What do you have there?" asked his mother.

"A piece of a wall," replied the child.

We know that a whole is sometimes perceived as more than the sum of its parts. In concept formation, wholeness takes on attributes, meanings or characteristics which may be quite apart from the components.

These may be dealt with without further reference to the whole. That is, we may engage in abstract thinking about attributes without specific reference to the origin of the abstracts.

When an accountant examines financial records, he deals mainly with a mathematical pattern and not necessarily with the innumerable business operations from which the pattern is derived. Yet, he can determine the financial conduct of the business without being aware of operational details. In a large business, the operational picture could not be determined at the level of individual operations. There would be so many of them that the examiner could not see the woods for the trees.

Somehow, operational events must be grouped and the groupings identified by symbols. The examiner then deals with the symbols, rather than the groupings or the components. In other words, he deals with the abstracts which represent actualities and not with the actualities themselves. Yet, the examiner remains aware of the relationship of the abstract with the actuality.

In using a map, we are aware that the map is a representation of a portion of the earth's surface from which it is derived perceptually. It is not actually a part of the earth's surface, yet we may use it as though it were. In navigation, the position of an object on the earth's surface can be located if its latitude and longitude are known. While we do not consider latitude and longitude as a physical part of the earth's surface, we apply them as though they were in navigation. We organize space and time into systems.

In concept formation, we reduce the variations in our environment so that we can "handle" them. We systematize large areas of the outer world and human activity and thus bring order out of chaos, organization out of disorganization and structure out of fragment. Once we have perceived the organization of parts in a whole, we can postulate the existence of the parts when some of them cannot be perceived at a given moment. Given the experienced totality of an object or situation, we can reconstruct the parts we cannot see.

Flip a coin. It's "heads." Without turning over the coin, we know that "tails" is on the other side. Then we may put the coin away and think about it a moment without reference to its physical structure. One of the attributes of the coin is value. It will exchange for a certain amount or kind of goods. It relates to other coins insofar as it may be a fraction or multiple of them and also insofar as it and they are part of a coinage system. In addition, it has a relationship to the coinage of other countries in a rate of exchange. Beyond this, it may have other values. It may be a rare coin, and have historical value. It may be the first coin earned in a new enterprise, and have sentimental value. It may be considered a "lucky" piece. In large, it may represent a culture, a period of history, a whole scheme of values.

All of these thoughts about the coin are not presented to the senses directly, but they are, nevertheless, real and they enter into the manner in which the coin may be used. Not only is our thinking about the coin based on characteristics which are observed in the present, but on relationships involving a similar coin experienced in the past. These past experiences may not only be utilized in an immediate perception of the coin, but also in conceiving of the coin as something more than a piece of metal alloy.

Concept derives from percept. Further, each process interacts with the other. The interaction may be so intimate that it cannot be, and should not be, dissociated. Concepts and percepts continuously modify each other. As the child matures, his view of the world changes with the acquisition of more and more perceptual data on which to form his concepts.

Concept formation draws on the whole time stream of experience. In a manner we do not fully understand, experiences undergone by the organism leave an impression, a mark, on the organism affecting future responses. This trace in the brain and central nervous system is the phenomenon we call memory. These traces of past experience which are retained may or may not be subject to conscious recall; but, whether conscious or not, they affect perceptual-conceptual activity and influence behavior.

The interaction of percept and concept accounts, in part, for the perceptually disabled child's difficulties in conceptual thinking. As concept formation proceeds, more materials are available for the enrichment of perception. And, as perception becomes enriched, it contributes more to concept. Either process may be depreciated by insufficiencies in the other.

The development of concepts serves to structure the perceptual world of the individual, so that percepts become more meaningful. This structuring, in turn, enables the individual to respond more adequately to his environment.

We have noted that the principal difficulty of the brain-injured child is that he does not make an adequate response to his environment in many respects. He may misperceive objects or situations and he may misinterpret them. Since the child's perceptual hold on reality may be rather tentative, the organization of perceptual experience he does achieve may tend to become rigid. This interferes with the development of new concepts. Concept formation requires the free manipulation of past percepts and where these are not firmly organized they cannot be manipulated freely. This may retard his intellectual development even though his intelligence may be normal. It may interfere with his academic progress, because learning is based on the formation of concepts through a concentration of perceptual experience.

Since his main difficulty is in organizing, much of the outer world which is systematized by the normal child remains patchy, and, therefore, incomprehensible, to the Other Child. Consequently, the brain-injured child is constantly exhibiting deficiencies in knowledge concerning his environment in some respects even though his knowledge may be adequate for his age in others. This unevenness in performance shows up in many brain-injured children of normal or near normal intelligence. It puzzles teachers who encounter the Other Child in the normal classroom in which the child seems intelligent enough but unaccountably deficient in some common knowledge. The "reluctance" of the Other Child to shift to more mature concepts may appear in his retention of what is called "animistic thinking" for a longer time than the normal child.

In its simplest form, animism represents a conceptual inability to dissociate living from nonliving material. We make deliberate use of this primitive thinking in modern culture. Airplanes and ships are "she," roads have "soft shoulders," the Mississippi is "Old Man River" and a hurricane is named "Diane."

To the young child, the table on which he bumps his head is a "bad" table and he may "kick it back." Even after he experiences the differences in animate and inanimate objects, the brain-injured child may persist in personifying inanimate objects longer because of his difficulty in rebuilding the earlier concept.

During his preschool years the normal child learns that not everything in his environment thinks and feels as he does. But while he is learning this, he often attributes motivations and behavior to inanimate objects. He feels personal resentment at the sky if the sun does not shine on his picnic-day. The toy hurt him and is a bad toy if his finger was scratched by it. His learning of the distinction between animate and inanimate is further complicated by our language which uses the same words for both. "Be careful, the knife will cut you" or "the swing will hit you," admonishes the mother. The young brain-injured child is literally confused if his mother asks "did you hurt your knee?" and may reply "No, the sidewalk scratched it." It takes him longer than it does for the normal child to discover how you play this game—that when you ask "did *you* hurt your knee" you are not suggesting a self-inflicted scratch but simply inquiring what happened.

As late as eight years of age a brain-injured child of near normal intelligence asked "why did I bump my head?" when he reached under the table to retrieve a fallen napkin. The question expressed his confusion about spatial relationships.

Often what appears to be animistic or even highly imaginative thinking is the child's use of his perceptual language—the only language he knows to describe events. He may ask about the lightning "why does the light go on there," not because he suspects someone turns it on but because he has no way to describe it except in terms of his own experiences. In some respects, the fantasy productions of the Other Child appear to be animistic explanations of objects and events the child cannot interpret in the normal way.

A seven-year-old boy tried to explain how Santa Claus was

tipped off about the behavior of children, since everybody was asleep when he was supposed to show up with his toys.

"Santa Claus started to climb down the chimney," said the boy, "but the chimney said, 'you can't come down here because that little boy has been a bad little boy.'"

The inability to organize experience into higher echelons of structure imposes a formidable handicap on the brain-injured child which is evident in much of his behavior—the inability to foresee consequences.

We know from past perceptions what is on the other side of the coin. We know, from past experience with similar coins, what a particular coin will buy without experiencing the purchase. We can relate the purchasing power of a coin to a commodity price structure.

The ability to predict, or foresee results, is conceptual. It relies on the application of past experience to what is presently being perceived. Our neighbors in the river bottoms can predict a flood when they see the river rising because they have experienced the cause and' effect before. When the cause and effect relationship has been established, either can be postulated from the other.

One aspect of the brain-injured child's dilemma is his frequent difficulty in relating cause and effect. He may not foresee the consequences of certain kinds of behavior, because the relationship of the behavior and its consequences in the past have been obscure. For this reason, punishment is often an inadequate way of correcting the Other Child's behavior. First, he may not be able to relate the punishment to the behavior which brought it on. And what has appeared to be misconduct to the parent, or punisher, may be the child's inability to respond appropriately to a situation imperfectly perceived or understood.

In normal mental development, the child begins to reason at about the age of eight. He then begins to see cause and effect relationships at the conceptual level. He can be reasoned with. When he is told that if he gets his shoes wet, he may catch a cold, he understands it, even though he may disregard the warning.

The brain-injured child may also commence to reason at the same age, but frequently in a different way. His reasoning may be "wrong." He may not be able to determine which aspects of situations produce certain effects, even though he may be able to understand causation.

A nine-year-old brain-injured child was told never to put his finger in an open electric socket because "it will shock you." "Can I put my toe in it?" he asked. Later, he heard his mother say on the telephone that she was "shocked" at hearing bad news about a friend. The child later reported: "Mommy got a shock today. She must have put her finger in the wall socket."

Much of the brain-injured child's confusion is reflected in language, the medium in which perceptual-conceptual structures are fixed. Early in life, the individual learns that naming or labeling experiences enables him to stabilize and manipulate them. Words are the tools of conception, but for the brain-injured child, they are often dull tools. Words help the normal person to "hold" percept and concept in the matrix of experience. The meanings of words become richer and more varied with conceptual development.

For the brain-injured child, whose concepts tend to be fairly rigid, the variable meanings of a word may be lost. A word may mean only one thing. It may stand for a single idea, irrespective of the context in which it is used. Moreover, the meaning of a word may be only partly comprehended and its use as a symbol only partially available. Consequently, the Other Child may have difficulty comprehending certain words, or may use them in the wrong context.

Brain-injured children frequently misuse words and appear to be talking nonsense, when actually their notion of the word meaning makes sense to them. A brain-injured boy of ten knew that the "train driver" was called an "engineer." A friend of the family asked him if he was going to study engineering when he grew up. "No," he responded, "I don't want to drive a train."

Sometimes, misuse of words results from perceptual difficulty in hearing a word. A thirteen year old girl referred to her sister's fiancé as "her finance." Not only was a perceptual error involved but the word, "finance," was empty of meaning.

Because of his tendency to cling to the structures he has already formed, the brain-injured child does not yield readily to the correction of perceptual or conceptual errors. Even when these are pointed out to him, he tends to perpetuate his mistakes. Restructuring is difficult for him. It requires tampering with structures which are not firmly held to begin with.

It is only with effort that the child progresses from one conceptual equilibrium to another. The progression tends to be slow. Sometimes, the child may regress to a lower level of mental activity, or a younger level. But when he does reach a new equilibrium, he holds it and is then ready to make further progress.

The brain-injured child may persist in mistakes in another way. The persistence relates to the tendency of many brain-injured children to repeat an activity once it is begun and to continue repeating it long after it has ceased to have any meaning or purpose. This kind of repetition is like a phonograph needle which becomes stuck in one groove of the record and keeps playing the same phrase over and over again. It is called perseveration.

Perseveration is the repetition of an activity without conscious will or purpose. It operates as though the whole nervous system, like the phonograph needle, had become stuck in the groove of a single response pattern. The child may continue to pound on the nail long after it has been driven into the wood. He may keep asking the same question, over and over again, even after it has been answered and he has understood the answer.

In arithmetic, perseveration may show up in counting. The child repeats the name of one number as he tries to move on to others. In writing, he tries to correct a letter he has formed incorrectly and through many erasures and new attempts continues to repeat his error.

The normal person may persevere at a task until it is finished. The brain-injured child goes further. He keeps at it after it is done. This is perseveration. Perseverance reflects the ability to structure and perform a task to completion, but in perseveration the child remains "stuck" and continues with his activity repetitiously.

There appear to be neurologic aspects to perseveration at the motor level of activity. Apparently, the energy of the child continues to seek an outlet in the continuation or repetition of the muscular movement, since the child cannot proceed at the moment to the organization of a new activity.

Brain-injured children frequently show perseverative behavior at the perceptual level, as we have indicated, and in concept formation, where older ideas are reiterated in place of new ones. In reading, the child may perseverate perceptually by repeating an error despite his own efforts and many attempts by the teacher to change it. He may perseverate conceptually by carrying over meanings to words where the meanings do not apply.

Perseveration appears to be a generalized disturbance of the entire neuromental system. However, normal persons may also perseverate especially under stress or when they are tired. Normal children may repeat acts in a way resembling the perseveration of the brain-injured child.

In the case of the normal child, the repetitive act is deliberate and gives satisfaction. The end result may even be highly positive. The child discovers modifications and experiments with new patterns as he learns the old ones. For the brain-injured child, there is often no satisfaction in the mechanical repetition of perseveration. Rather than being led through chance or deliberate modifications of the activity to a variation of it, his behavior becomes automatic and stereotyped or deteriorates.

Concept formation in the brain-injured child may be disturbed in several ways: by the child's perceptual disability, which interferes with the acquisition and organization of data; by his difficulty in manipulating abstracts and reorganizing percepts and by the resulting rigidity of his concepts.

One of the questions most frequently asked about brain injury is whether damage to particular portions of the brain specifically produces perceptual or conceptual malfunctioning. Certain brain functions do appear to be highly localized. Interpretation of sensory data seems to occur in certain portions of the cortex. Damage to these specific areas affects the ability to organize these data. However, much of the brain does not appear to show such close correspondence with psychological processes. Rather, it seems to function in terms of a broad matrix for the interaction of many activities at once. We think of the brain as being an interacting network in which processes are operating all the time, with interaction between the processes occurring on a wide base. If this is so, it would appear that damage to the brain may result in a generalized disturbance of the processes of interaction. It is not a single process which is disturbed, but the integration and interaction of processes.

Malfunctioning of the perceptual-conceptual processes tends to produce abnormal behavior. It is through his behavior and his learning difficulties that the plight of the brain-injured child becomes visible.

When we consider that the continual interplay of perceptual-conceptual processes is involved in every response we make to every situation, we can appreciate the difficulties of the brain-injured child in finding equilibrium in a highly organized and complex culture. Frequently, he does not find it himself. Unless he is shown how, he remains a disturbed and unhappy child.

CHAPTER IV

LANGUAGE: Thinking Is Communicating

An important criterion of the child's development is his ability to use language. The degree of language ability is commonly equated with intelligence. A deficiency in language, however, may not necessarily reflect a deficiency in intelligence. It does reflect a handicap, but the handicap may be physiological or cultural, as well as intellectual, in origin.

Language disturbances in children arise principally as the result of defects in the sensory apparatus by which sounds are received and transmitted to the brain or as the result of perceptual disability. A deaf child is prevented from learning to use language in the normal way because he cannot hear it. The brain-injured child is handicapped in the development of language, even though his hearing is normal, because he does not perceive adequately what he hears.

Brain injury may result in the failure of language to develop, in the loss of language after it has developed or in a lack of ability to use language adequately because of disturbances in perception and concept formation.

In this book, we are concerned with language in its broadest definition as a communicative channel of thought. While language is commonly identified with speech, we know that speech is merely the vocal expression of language. Some cultures, such as the Amerind, have a highly developed sign language. Deaf persons use signs to communicate language to each other.

A person who loses the use of speech organs after language has developed does not necessarily lose language. Speech depends on language, but language does not depend on speech.

As the symbolic expression of experiences, language is used inwardly, to communicate with self, and outwardly to communicate with others. Internally, we use language to anchor a wide range of experiences and ideas. These are organized into a symbol, or a series of symbols, and may thus be manipulated in thinking or transmitted to convey thinking to others.

Externally, we use language as a means of relating to other persons. Through language, social organization, involving the interaction of individuals, becomes possible. Thus, we think of language as the means by which individual thinking is organized and as the means by which society is organized and perpetuated.

Words are the principal symbols used to carry thought as thought is transmuted into patterns of sound or visual stimuli. But in the realm of technology and science, words become inadequate and are replaced by mathematical symbols representing a further condensation of experience and ideas.

We consider language as a noninstinctive means of communication available only to human beings. Language may be attributed poetically to animals and insects which communicate and respond to signals. But the capacity for language symbolization exists only in the human neuromental organization.

While the capacity for developing language is inherent in human beings, the use of language has to be learned. It does not exist, full grown, in the inexperienced mind of the infant. Language is the product of the experienced mind of the adult. The child learns the language of his culture, but some languages are harder to learn than others, a factor which bears on the plight of the brain-injured child in America.

Some linguists have made a strong case for the theory that the English language presents special difficulties to the child—difficulties which do not exist, or are less troublesome, in other European languages.

Consequently, it appears that the American child must exert greater perceptual and intellectual effort in learning English than the Italian child in learning Italian, the French child in learning French and the German child in learning German.

English is not a pure language, but an amalgamation of Greek, Latin, French and Germanic language elements. Much of the imagery associated with root words, which lend the modern word color and content, have been lost in English, but retained in the Romance and Germanic languages.

As an example, consider the word, "language," itself. It derives from the common French noun, *la langue*, which means both "tongue" and "language" and which is rooted in the Latin word, *lingua*, also meaning "tongue" or "language." The conceptual meaning of *la langue* in terms of "language" is suggested to the French child in terms of the perceptual reference to "tongue." The French word has a recognizable relationship in sound and structure to the Latin root. The English speaking child is not so fortunate. While the words "tongue" and "language" are used synonymously, they are different words with different origins. "Tongue" derives from the Old Teutonic *tungen* and the Middle English *tunge*. It has no visual or auditory relationship to "language."

Persons who can speak two languages are not "two-tongued," but "bi-lingual" and an expert in many tongues is a "linguist." Thus, perceptual origins of many English words are lost to the child because they exist in other languages. More frequently, these origins, which serve to fortify and enrich meanings, have persisted in the Romance and Germanic languages.

Because of its compound origin, the English language contains many discrepancies in auditory and visual representations. The "K" sound may appear visually as "ch" in chemical, "c" in cat or "k" in kitchen. The "ch" symbol may be sounded differently, as in "which," "chute" or "ache." For the brain-injured child, English presents perceptual difficulties which are hardly encountered to such a degree in other European languages.

Aside from the comparative difficulties of various languages, language development appears consistent and typical among normal children. The first sound which issues from the newborn infant is the birth cry. It is followed in the first few months by such reflexive sounds as grunts, coos, gurgles, hiccoughs, snorts and wails. About the fifth or sixth month, the child begins to experiment with sound production. He babbles. While the child may reproduce some phonetic elements of speech in his babbling, these appear to be accidental rather than consciously imitative. He is interested in making sounds for their own sake.

At about twelve months, the child will echo a sound pattern produced by those around him. During this period, his sound production sets up a circular reaction. When he echoes a syllable he hears from others, he stimulates the need within himself to respond to the sound patterns he has produced. Since the syllable previously produced is available for response, he responds to it by repeating it.

In this way, the child establishes a feedback system in which the production of speech sounds becomes associated with his auditory perception of the sounds. He begins to perceive the linkage of these functions. And he commences to be able to control the sounds he produces.

Echoic responses form a significant part of the child's utterances up to about thirty months of age. They set up the essential motor basis for future speech. The first words usually are repeated monosyllables, such as "ma ma," "da da" or "bye bye." They are used to apply to persons or things he has perceived in his environment. The objects or individuals represented by these words may not be strongly structured. To the young child, a "tick-tock" may be any round, shiny object, not necessarily a watch, and "da da" may apply to any adult male. The name words are not specific because the perceptions to which the words apply are not highly differentiated.

As the child's perceptual ability increases, and he becomes able to differentiate and compare, his labels become more specific and more consistent in their reference to persons or objects. As he acquires vocabulary, the child begins to accompany his actions with words. He uses language in monologue to express his own activity. At this stage, he may not use language to communicate with others, but with self. The function of monologues seems to be the fixing of percepts as the child moves from one perceptual experience to another. The child uses language to maintain the orderly arrangement of his perceptions.

For the young child, language is a means of holding perceptions and thus organizing or stabilizing the environment. How many times has one heard a child saying, "that's a doggie, that's a doggie" whether anyone is present or not? Is the child trying to communicate with someone? Or does he seem to be talking to himself?

In his early use of language, the child seems to be vocalizing his percepts, as though trying to structure them in words. His language records his developing perceptions. A "doggie" becomes a "big doggie" or "my doggie" as his awareness of relationship grows.

Some of the child's effort to organize his perceptual world is revealed in the assertiveness of his speech. His assertions may not involve other persons. He is simply declaiming to himself.

Early in life, the child learns that certain sounds elicit a response from others. In this way, he finds he can communicate his needs. Later, he learns to copy the sound patterns used by those who respond to him and to use these patterns in seeking a response from others.

When he has gained enough perceptual experience, and sufficient language, he finds that he is able to acquire percepts from others as these are communicated to him through language. In this way, he can enlarge his perceptual world with experiences he has not actually undergone.

The young child's communication does not involve concept. His learning through language proceeds on the perceptual level. His use of language is couched in the perceptual frame of reference. The meanings he attaches to words relate to perceptual experience.

Consequently, when the child begins asking, "why," he usually means, "what." A four year-old boy when admonished not to "cry like a baby" asks "why am I a baby?" He may be trying to pin down what differences exist between himself and a baby. A child who has learned the names of numbers up to seven asks, "who comes after seven?"

The child who asks, "why is the sky blue?" does not expect a scientific explanation. He may be seeking more perceptual detail about the sky. Essentially, he is asking "what" about the sky. This does not make his questions any easier to answer, but sometimes providing more description about the thing he is questioning serves to fill in the "what" about it.

The child's use of language parallels his perceptual and, later, his conceptual development. If the child has a perceptual disability, it would be expected to show up in his use of language. Our experience with brain-injured children shows that it does. Further, if percepts are unstable or poorly organized, the language representations may tend to be inadequate or inconsistent.

A nine year old boy asked, "what is an urr?" No one had ever heard of an "urr" and the boy was accused of making it up. This distressed him. He insisted he had seen an "urr." Where?

"It's in the pink bull book," he said. "I saw it." The pink bull book was a child's edition of "Ferdinand the Bull." The boy turned the pages until he came to a picture.

"There," he said triumphantly. "There is an urr." He pointed to the matador. When the word was first read to him, he had perceived it only in terms of the last syllable.

After her vacation, an eight year old girl reported she had seen a "skinx." It was made out of stone, it had big ears and she saw it in a picture book.

"That was the Sphinx," her teacher corrected.

"Yes," said the girl. "The skinx."

Inadequate use of language sometimes results in apparent irrelevancies. On an overcast day, a nine year old girl reported she saw the sun shining. Obviously, she could not have seen the sun shining because it had been cloudy all day. Where was the sun shining? The girl pointed to a feeble ribbon of light filtering through the clouds. She was unable to verbalize the distinction between this and the bright sunshine of a cloudless day.

Since language is largely the basis of interpersonal relationships between human beings, the child's relationships with others tends to be adversely affected by language deficiency. The brain-injured child may not only fail to communicate adequately, but he may misconstrue what is communicated to him and thus may fail to respond to what is said to him in the expected way.

Moreover, the Other Child frequently says the "wrong" thing

in situations in which he lacks the appropriate words or misconstrues the situation. His erratic use of language creates an endless array of interpersonal difficulties for him. These bewilder and tend to disorganize him because he does not comprehend their cause.

Adults notice that the child "says silly things" and other children report that "he talks funny." A boy who persisted in talking back to his parents and teachers was admonished about this. He asked: "Is it all right if I talk back, 'hello' and 'thank you'?" The boy had assigned one meaning to the phrase, "talk back." To him it meant reply. It was apparent that he did not perceive the connotation of discourtesy or impudence in the phrase.

The child's ability to use and respond to language depends on the degree to which his perceptual experiences have been organized. Until he is seven or eight years old, the child does not have a permanent group of concepts which he can manipulate freely. It is difficult for him to modify them to incorporate the views of an adult. It is more effective to show the child rather than to attempt only to reason with him in influencing his behavior.

As his perceptual development proceeds, the child begins to differentiate his perceptions. He extracts what is pertinent and relegates into the background what is irrelevant. His words then represent the differentiated perception.

In this growth, words do not simply represent an object, but refer to the characteristics of the object. The words now become symbols which refer not only to objects but to their characteristics, uses and ways in which the objects are thought about.

As the child broadens his definitions, his words reflect concepts. The process of conceptual language has begun. As this process develops, the child enters the framework of adult reality and commences to use language as adults use it.

With the development of conceptualization, the child becomes able to abstract similarities from a number of perceptions and manipulate them in his thinking. He now works with abstractions which he organizes into new wholes—or concepts.

The process of concept formation usually begins in the seventh or eighth year. He commences to use conceptual rather than perceptual language. As this ability develops, he becomes susceptible to being influenced by language since at this point he can accept the substitution of symbols for experience in modifying his behavior. When he is able to manipulate abstracts, through the symbols pertaining to them, he can reason.

In general, we believe that conceptualization appears when the organism reaches a stage of biologic development which makes it possible, irrespective of the state of development of specific abilities.

We have used the term biologic age, rather than chronologic age, since the rate of physiologic development varies. In any age group, one finds a wide range of individual differences in maturation. The brain-injured child may or may not begin to conceptualize at the same biologic age as the normal child. Because of his difficulties in organizing concepts, however, he tends to cling to perceptual language longer. He has difficulty developing language as symbolism because to do so requires the organization of many facets of experience into a manageable unit. It is in organizing that the brain-injured child has particular difficulty.

The Other Child's perceptual confusion in figure and ground organization impairs his ability to abstract the essential elements of perceived experience and combine them into adequate concepts. If the child cannot organize experience adequately, he cannot represent it adequately through language. Moreover, the language representations may be poorly structured, so that the meanings of words he both uses and hears from others are not quite clear to him.

We find that a brain-injured child may have a large vocabulary, but at the same time tend to use words only in terms of their specific meanings. While he might use a general name, he might fail to grasp the generality implied in the word. A symbol may mean less to him than to the normal child. His comprehension of the symbol may vacillate, as first one element, then another, of his incomplete concepts assumes foreground priority. Because of his tendency to avoid restructuring experience, the brain-injured child's use of language frequently lags in relation to his biologic age. He may use words and phrases characteristic of the child younger than himself.

When he was five, R. listened to a story about a toy mender. At age ten, when the crossbar on his kite broke, R. talked of taking the kite to "the toy mender." When the inappropriateness of the term was explained to him, R. said, "I know. Toy menders are only in books." Even at twelve, R. would vacillate between referring to birthday presents, such as a watch or a table radio, as "toys" and referring to them as "gifts." The older generalization was easier for him, although he was aware that a watch and radio were not toys.

At school, R. was ridiculed when he said that after school he was going home to play. He learned it was more acceptable in his age group to say he was going to "play ball" or "monkey around." Under social pressure, he was compelled to revise his use of words.

While the vocabulary of the brain-injured child may be as large as that of the normal child, the former has considerably more difficulty in combining words so that they reflect experiences.

J. would attend the movies regularly every Saturday afternoon, but he was at a loss when asked to tell what he saw. He was unable to describe the plot of the movie. Instead, he would relate: "Oh, there was this part where a man got his foot stuck in a bucket." When asked whether he liked the movie better than the one he had seen the previous week, he would reply without hesitation. It was easier for him to relate his reaction to the movie than to restructure it in language.

In grammar, the brain-injured child may have particular difficulty because grammar, again, is organization. Grammatical confusion is conspicuous among brain-injured children, even those from homes in which correct grammar is habitually used. While the child may have no difficulty memorizing the rules of grammar, he may be unable to apply them, since the applications may not be clear to him.

The irregularity of the English language poses a particular handicap in communication to the brain-injured child. Not only is he subject to the ordinary difficulty in learning irregular constructions but he is also confused by words which sound alike but refer to different things and by words which mean the same thing but have no phonetic relationship. In America, this difficulty is compounded because the child resides in a culture which has little gesture language to reinforce the meanings of words. Gestures provide a visual aid for the child by which he can check his auditory perceptions.

But in the average household, gestures are not available to help him determine the emotional as well as the semantic content of speech. He may tend to use words with high emotional content in situations where there is no emotional context and vice versa.

A particular problem of the adolescent brain-injured boy is a tendency to use profane or visceral words indiscriminately. This apparent lack of inhibition may actually reflect the boy's inability to structure social situations and make adequate responses to them. The boy may lack awareness of the appropriateness or inappropriateness of certain words in particular situations.

Involved in this problem is the brain-injured child's difficulty in assessing the attitudes of others toward himself. One problem in making such an assessment may be language deficiency. Language is one means by which the evaluation of the individual's performance in society is fed back to him. The feedback when it is perceived has a tendency to modify behavior. To achieve the modification, it is necessary to reorganize behavior structures, to remodel them, so to speak. Because of his reluctance to tamper with already shaky structures, the brain-injured child finds it extremely hard to "change his ways" even when he understands the necessity for doing so.

His rigidity in attitudes and behavioral responses give the appearance that he is oblivious to the opinion of others and insensitive to criticism. Experience with many brain-injured children indicates this apparent insensitivity is a product of the child's difficulty in grasping the attitudes of others through language. Actually, the brain-injured child tries harder to win approval than his normal brother or sister, because he has a special need to stabilize his relationships with other persons in an environment which frequently appears quite unstable to him.

Difficulties in the use of language are called aphasia. The term has been applied principally to adults who have lost the ability to use language after it has grown to its full expression as a communicative channel of thought.

We identify the aphasia of children by another term, oligophasia, meaning a deficit in language or the lack of its development. In many respects, it appears that this condition is different from the condition in adults. In general, we find three types of oligophasia in brain-injured children.

If the language difficulty is primarily a result of disturbance in auditory perception, the child may be said to have receptive oligophasia. Figure and ground relation of auditory elements cannot be recognized clearly. The percept is disorganized and fragmented, as in "what is an urr?"

If the language disturbance appears in the formation of speech patterns and the transmission of them through the organs of speech, the condition is called expressive oligophasia.

The third type of oligophasia we call central oligophasia. It is a disorder in symbolization so that language cannot be evolved. Some words may exist, but even if they can be used, they cannot serve as references for concepts.

The treatment of oligophasia must take into account the fact of brain damage, with resulting perceptual-conceptual disorganization. From this viewpoint, an attempt is made to educate the child in terms of improving perceptual-conceptual organization along with specific attention to the language deficit.

Frequently, a brain-injured child cannot seem to understand the speech of someone he is not familiar with. He keeps saying "what?" "what?" His confusion increases if his failure to understand is misconstrued as a hearing impediment and the person speaking to him raises his voice.

When the child says, "what?" he does not necessarily mean "I don't hear you." He may mean, "I don't understand you." In this respect, he reacts like a person hearing bad news for the first time. The person is unable to "believe" the bad news and says, "what?", not because he didn't hear it, but frequently because it involves restructuring or reorientation which are aided by redundancy.

When a person raises his voice to repeat to the brain-injured child, the increase in volume may introduce an emotional element which tends to cancel out the effect of redundancy. The child may be aided to comprehend instructions, for example, if they are given after an initial preparation and repeated, if necessary, calmly and slowly.

The instruction should, as far as possible, structure the situation for the child. They should also be given chronologically, first things first. A boy who is asked to shovel snow is more likely to respond immediately to the instruction if he is told: (1) There is a lot of snow on the walk; (2) put on your hat, coat and gloves (3) get the snow shovel off the back porch (4) shovel the snow off the walk. When he has perceived the structure of what he is asked to do, he does not ask, "what?"

As we have indicated, gesturing helps the child to comprehend language. Gesturing has become a lost art in this country in everyday speech, but it can often convey the nuances of language more effectively than speech.

A generation ago, grammar school children were occasionally treated to the performances of Chief Evergreen Tree on the school assembly circuit. The Chief was a venerable showman and highly regarded by school principals. He not only imparted information to the pupils but he was entertaining as well, a combination not often achieved in the school assembly programs of the day. The Chief would demonstrate some Indian sign language gestures. Then he would proceed to use them to illustrate his talk. One of the signs was the wiggling of two fingers on the hand as the hand descended from the mouth. This denoted a crooked, or lying, tongue. Then the Chief would tell a tall story exaggerating his prowess. Some of the more perceptive children would become aware of the exaggeration and show their amusement. But it was not until the end of the tale, when the Chief would give the sign for lying tongue, that the whole assembly would burst into laughter.

Gestures and pantomime help enrich the communication reception of the brain-injured child, as they enrich the understanding of everyone. The performances of the actor, the evangelist and the old style politician are rich in gestures. Performers know that gestures are part of language and help communicate it as a supplement to speech.

It is not unusual to find that some brain-injured children are highly verbal. They seem to have good expressive language facility but some of this verbal facility may be imitative. The child may use words without being certain of their content. The percepts or concepts which the words represent may not be firmly evolved.

In highly verbal brain-injured children, there is often a gap between the apparent ability to use language and its comprehension. There may also be a wide discrepancy between talking and doing. The child's actual performance may be on a lower level than his ability to talk about it.

Such discrepancies in the performance of the brain-injured child are characteristic of his disability.

Much has been accomplished in special education to improve the Other Child's use of language. Speech correction may be an important part of the therapy. But the brain-injured child's language difficulties are frequently a manifestation of malfunctioning of the perceptual-conceptual processes which language represents. It is on this basis, we believe, that special education can effectively approach the Other Child's language problems.

CHAPTER V

BEHAVIOR: Action and Reaction

When we speak of behavior, we do not necessarily limit the meaning of the term to the manner in which an individual conducts himself in relation to others. Rather, we consider behavior as the totality of responses the individual makes to his environment. In this light, it is evident that inadequacy of response to environmental stimuli leads to inadequate behavior, so that the individual does not cope successfully with his environment. This essentially is the plight of the brain-injured child. He frequently finds himself unable to behave in such a way as to meet environmental demands.

In considering the behavior difficulties of the brain-injured child, we emphasize certain characteristics which relate to brain injury and which distinguish this child as otherwise. We view these behavior manifestations as physiologic rather than emotional in origin insofar as they appear to be the consequence of neuromental malfunctioning. But it is also evident that emotional disturbance intensifies these physiologically-based behavioral anomalies as well as increasing the frequency of their appearance. The most conspicuous of these difficulties are hyperkinesis (hyperactivity), distractibility (short attention span), disinhibition (impulsivity), inflexibility (including perseveration) and emotional instability. All or some of them may show up in the behavior of the brain-injured child.

To parents and teachers, the hyperkinesis and splintered attention in all of their variants are often the most exhausting and annoying. The emotional lability, including as it does anger out-

61

bursts and catastrophic reactions to frustration, is most baffling because of the magnitude of the reaction in proportion to the triggering stimulus.

In addition to these particular disorders, the brain-injured child may show an inability to conform to the behavioral patterns of his age group because he does not perceive the patterns correctly and is unsure of what is expected of him.

The behavior difficulties which appear specific to brain injury account for only a part of the Other Child's behavior. It is subject, too, to the emotional disturbances that may afflict any child. However, it is not within the scope of this book to discuss the emotional disorders of children.

We can say only that the brain-injured child's physiologically based behavior anomalies may result in emotional disturbance inasmuch as they increase his environmental difficulties and influence the attitudes of others toward him. Since his behavior is more difficult than that of other children in the family, he is corrected more often and more vehemently; it is not surprising if he begins to feel unfairly treated and resentful because of these feelings. It is probable that some of the Other Child's emotional problems can be eased or avoided if the nature of his "misbehavior" is understood.

Descriptions by parents of the course of the brain-injured child's development often contain references to hyperactivity or, as it is often called, hyperkinesis. Often, already as an infant the brain-injured child is less placid, less contented and less easily scheduled than his normal siblings. Many such children are more restless in their cribs, sleep lightly and irregularly, and cry fretfully although there seems to be no observable reason for their discontent. Mothers often find that their brain-injured child is not as easy to cuddle as other children and that instead of relaxing in her arms he remains tense. Sudden sensory stimulation produces an overflow of response. A loud noise or jerk may cause a strong startle reaction and the child may begin to cry from the uncomfortable sensations which were aroused. Even the turning on or off of a light may have a similar disquieting effect.

Not all brain-injured children show these evidences of poor central nervous system integration during their infancy, how-

ever. Many are less active than normal children and less responsive to stimuli. It is not until they begin to crawl or walk that
many become hyperactive. Mothers report that the child was
seldom still, that he resisted their efforts to keep him in a high
chair or in the play pen even for short periods of time, and that
whenever he moved he ran rather than walked. His exploratory
behavior appears random or aimless rather than purposive, in
part because of the pell-mell pace at which it is pursued, in part
because of the quick and cursory interest devoted to objects
within the environment. As soon as a stimulus is identified the
child is ready to respond to another, generally quite unrelated
to the first. His waking moments consist of a stream of mosaics
which by his nature he is compelled to note and identify but
which his brain injury prevents him from organizing into a pattern of relationships: It is as though the sense organs, which
should be the channel to the higher processes of perception and
conception, are instead a pathway to the motor system. This is
not difficult to understand if one remembers that the motor system by virtue of its organization is constructed so that stimuli
from the world outside can touch triggers which set it into action. Even in adults many motor acts occur within a split second
of the stimulating situation, without our conscious volition. A
falling cup is caught almost before the mind has grasped the
situation, or a car is avoided by quickly jumping to the side, and
only after the act has been completed does the mind comprehend fully what has occurred.

With the combination of neurological maturation and the persistent efforts of the social group to instill control, the hyperactivity of the brain-injured child diminishes as he grows older. In
nursery school it may still be a rather serious problem. By the
time the child is of school age it may be manifest as a greater
restlessness or a drive to move about more than the average child
of the same age. In the usual classroom the teacher finds that
the brain-injured child is more apt to engage in restless motor
activity such as shuffling his feet, tapping with a pencil, twist-
ing and squirming on his chair, getting up and down to adjust
his clothing and so on, with no motive of drawing attention to
himself but simply because he must respond to his inner and

outer environment with motor activity. The child is often over-active in the classroom; he goes more frequently than necessary to the reading shelf, he stops on his way to look at pictures on the bulletin board, he comes to the teacher with little bits of information, he requests permission to go to the washroom and so on through a host of activities too numerous to mention. The child may even become rather skillful in inventing pretexts for activity and thus be able to fulfill his need for movement without seriously offending his teacher. In fact, a remark often made by the teacher is that "he's not a bad child but I can't get him to sit still and really pay attention."

One of the most important achievements of the child is the development of purposeful behavior for himself and the ability to share actively in the purposeful behavior of others, by accepting their goals as his own. This is the foundation of social growth. It is also the wellspring which the teacher uses in guiding her pupils to mastery of one new skill after another.

For the normal person, purposeful activity represents a co-ordination of experience, evaluation of the possibilities and results of various responses and the structuring of a goal that the individual wants to reach. All of these elements of goal-directed activity involve perceptual and conceptual organization. It is in the realm of organization that the brain-injured child encounters his greatest difficulty. It is not surprising to find, therefore, that he appears to be deficient, in many instances, in the ability to formulate and carry out a plan. His purposeful activity is characterized by vagueness and incompleteness. His goals are not only inadequately structured, but his evaluation of the situations he encounters in an effort to reach them tends to be faulty. For this reason, much of the activity of the brain-injured child may appear to be purposeless and many of his actions without apparent meaning. He may have an objective in mind, but it is so poorly conceived and operationally so difficult for him that he cannot carry it out.

A boy of 11 decided he wanted to put up a tent in his back yard. He was given an old blanket and advised to drape it over a clothesline. He followed the advice and sometime later he was found sitting under the edges of the blanket which he had simply hung on the clothesline.

In normal perception, the individual segregates the foreground figure and the background. In doing so, he has accomplished two things. He focuses his attention on the figure but at the same time he is aware not only of the relationship between figure and ground but conscious also of their relation to himself.

A motorist is driving along the highway in Sunday traffic. He is aware, or should be, of other autos in front of him, beside him and behind him. From time to time, he checks their position relative to his own by glancing from side to side and at the rear-view mirror. Now he passes a scene where a traffic policeman has stopped a car and is giving the driver a ticket. If he is overly distracted by the scene, he is immediately in danger of losing track of his position relative to that of other moving vehicles on the crowded roadway. And then, of course, he places himself in danger of a collision. The sophisticated motorist is aware of this. If he is momentarily distracted, he swings back quickly to the primary focus of his attention, which is relating himself to the traffic pattern. He relegates such distractions as the traffic ticket scene, low flying airplanes, etc. into the background. His behavior in traffic is adequate.

The brain-injured child has difficulty in perceiving the relationship of figure and ground, which is essentially a process of organization. He has difficulty in relating these elements to himself. Consequently, his perception of physical structures and of situations tends to be fragmented. When he cannot pattern an array of stimuli into a comprehensive whole, he cannot tell which are significant to him and which are not. It is not surprising, then, that he may not focus his attention on the configuration which would normally be perceived as in the foreground. Background stimuli or stimuli extraneous to the foreground figure may have the same power to compel his attention as the figure. When this occurs, his attention proceeds from one detail of the pattern to another. It is unlikely that he will become aware of the foreground figure in its relationship to the background until it is pointed out to him. This can be observed in the brain-injured child's response to pictures. For example, given a picture which shows in the foreground a group of people reading a newspaper, the brain-injured child may neglect this foreground entirely and say that he sees a lady by the house—a tiny figure included only to add detail to the scene.

The child's attraction to details can be observed in the manner in which he responds to his environment. He is the one who observes the missing button on the visitor's shirt, the thread on the sleeve, the speck on the page, and so on. If he has a hangnail or the smallest cut he may find it nearly impossible to disregard it and to give his full attention to a lesson or a game. A loose button, the end of a thread, a torn label, the unpasted corner of a picture will be fingered and fussed with until it can be repaired or until it is removed.

The brain-injured child's difficulty in perceptual organization has the effect of increasing the power of extraneous stimuli to capture his attention. Even though he may perceive the relation of figure and ground, his "hold" on the pattern may be insecure. It may vacillate for him. It may slip away from him. The vacillation and confusion to which he is subject in structuring experience have a profound effect on his behavior. They diminish his ability to complete tasks, particularly when the manner in which the task is to be performed is weakly structured and the goal indefinite. We describe this frequent shifting of attention and deficit of purposeful activity as "distractibility." Like the hyperkinesis, it is a product of brain pathology rather than a reaction to emotional tensions.

In school, the teacher observes that the child is not paying attention to the lesson unless she is standing over him, helping by her presence or by reminders of the goal to narrow his attention. In a regular classroom of 30 to 40 pupils, this procedure is obviously impossible.

Attracted by a noise behind him, the child turns around in his seat to find its source. While he looks for it, another child drops a pencil and he must watch until the pencil is retrieved. Still another child gets up to speak to the teacher and he is attracted to this new activity. Meanwhile, a truck passes the classroom and he strains to watch it as long as it remains in view. From his work at the blackboard, his attention is drawn to the sound of footsteps in the hall. He may become entranced by the ticking of the classroom clock. He seems to be unable to complete anything he is given to do.

His teacher may refer to this behavior as "limited span of attention," a phrase which seems dubious in reference to the brain-injured child. If the "span of attention" is deemed "too limited," the child may be regarded as "not ready" for schooling. The term "readiness," as it is frequently used by school authorities, seems to refer to a level of neuromental development in the normal child which enables him to acquire educational experience and adjust to a conventional classroom situation. Normally, this developmental level is reached at about age six, although many normal children reach it sooner and many later. When a child is said to be "not ready" for a formal learning experience, it is usually assumed that he will become "ready" in time. But time alone does not make the brain-injured child "ready." He must be helped to become "ready" by a program of special instruction which takes into account the effects of the child's perceptual handicap in shaping his behavior. Some methods by which this can be done will be described in a later chapter.

We do not feel that the child's "limited span of attention" means that he is inattentive, rather he is overattentive to irrelevancies. He does not focus on the significant element of experience because his attention is attracted to many elements. He attends to numerous stimuli in his sensory field, a jack of all trades, but master of none. Attention-wise, he is unable to specialize when a situation is so loosely structured for him that he cannot find in it a central focus or pattern. All of the elements in the situation are equally significant and relevant for him and therefore deserving of his attention. If the problem of structuring the classroom situation, or his lessons, is made simpler for him, the brain-injured child's distractability decreases. To state it another way, his "span of attention" increases.

In the special class for the brain-injured child, the number of possible distractions is reduced. Material is presented to him at whichever level he can successfully organize it. If he is not ready to learn academically, experiences which promote readiness are provided. Such an approach enables the child to organize his experiences. When he is able to do this, his distractibility comes under his own control. While it may not disappear, it no longer disrupts him from completing his task. He can attend to the distracting event, perceive its meaning to his satisfaction and return to his lesson without reminder, coaxing or urging. In short, he becomes a pupil. He is able to make academic progress and to realize the potential for learning which still lies within him. In this way, the child's responses are made more adequate. His behavior changes. His relationship to teachers and parents improves.

One thinks of the term, "inhibition," as the suppression of certain responses in a situation where they would be inappropriate. Disinhibition describes the failure to suppress the inappropriate or inadequate response.

Put in another way, inhibition involves not only the suppression of some responses but also their suppression in favor of the most appropriate response the individual can make. In a situation in which a number of responses are possible, the element of selection is indicated. Thus, the individual selects the responses which he considers the most adequate. In the classroom, the teacher asks a question which several children believe they can answer. The manner in which the class is conducted requires that volunteers must seek recognition from the teacher by raising their hands. When one is recognized, the others are required to subside.

The disinhibited child, however, does not conform to this procedure. He may not go through the procedure for recognition, but may call out, "I know, I know" or he may blurt out the answer. Either he may not perceive the procedural formula for recognition or he may impulsively bypass it. In either case, he does not select the appropriate response in terms of the classroom situation while inhibiting the inappropriate ones.

On the other hand, the individual may find himself in situations in which disinhibited responses may not only be tolerated but expected. At a political rally, at which emotional appeals are made to the audience by the orator, fervent cries of agreement from individuals reinforce the situation and are considered appropriate. Heckling and shouts of disapproval conform to the structure of the rally.

In either case, there is a selectivity of response in relation to the situation. When the individual makes consistently inappropriate responses either in kind or in degree he appears to be disinhibited. Selection of response entails the evaluation of the situation in terms of past experience. It involves a high level of perceptual and conceptual activity. While only one response is made, a number may have been considered and repressed in the process of selection.

It has been indicated that the brain-injured child fails to develop as wide a variety of responses to stimuli as the normal child. Consequently, it would appear that his range of selection is more limited. He may repeat the same response in a variety of situations irrespective of its appropriateness. Or, perceiving only one aspect of a situation, he may respond to it rather than to the total situation.

Additionally, he may not be able to control the intensity of his response and may over-react. Thus, if a group laughs, he laughs louder and longer than his fellows, if cheering is acceptable he shouts, if bodily expression is used to show enthusiasm he not only jumps up and down and waves his arms but he pummels his companion or grabs him excitedly in a tight embrace.

Frequently, the child's poor controls and his inability to forsee clearly the consequences of an action lead him to act impulsively or disinhibitedly and then regret the action. On the playground, the child may be so intent on obtaining the ball that he wrests it away from a playmate while roughly pushing him to the ground. When the playmate is angered or tearful, the "culprit" is sincerely regretful, solicitous of the hurt and anxious to restore good feelings once again.

A normally intelligent brain-injured boy of nine years impulsively snipped a hole in the sweater-sleeve of his teacher and was mortified after he had done it. He had no explanation for the act, and could only say he couldn't help it and didn't mean to do it. The scissors in his hand and the teacher's sleeve within close range impelled him to action without the restraining effect of the anticipation of her amazement and his shame.

The impulsiveness of many brain-injured children makes them more liable to traffic accidents and other injuries than normal children. In his headlong dash to cross a street or to retrieve his ball, the impulsive brain-injured child is functionally blind to or unperceptive of the dangers involved. He often lacks fear and is heedless of the consequences of his behavior. He lacks caution because he cannot anticipate and evaluate.

This is in direct contrast to the behavior of many brain-injured children who are not impulsive or particularly disinhibited except under stimulating circumstances. Such children learn caution as a method of adaptation to their perceptual inadequacies and defective perceptuo-motor integration. They descend stairs carefully, holding on to the railing; if children are playing a jumping game, they jump from the second step rather than the third or fourth; they avoid climbing high or jumping on or off playground equipment. Although they are awkward in motion and are clumsy, and to the uninitiated observer in danger of falling, the caution they have learned as an adaptive response usually keeps them from serious injury. An exception is this child's behavior with equipment such as sleds, wagons and bicycles. The child is unprepared by his poor visuo-motor apparatus to make the rapid perceptions and adjustments required under the new conditions of increased speed.

As with hyperkinesis and distractibility, the development of inhibitory controls increases with maturation and learning. As the child's perception of the world he lives in is filled in with organized experiences, he learns to assess situations more appropriately and to hold back responses which are inappropriate.

The children themselves, as they mature, learn to recognize signs of impending loss of control and develop means of preventing it. An 11 year old boy would become overly excited and consequently restless and silly whenever his parents entertained a small group of guests. He learned to excuse himself to either one of his parents whenever he recognized the symptoms of mounting tension by saying "I'm beginning to feel fussy, may I go to my room?" In the quiet of his own room he would play his records, look at books or read until he felt composed again and could rejoin the company.

Other children with serious difficulty in a given school subject will ask to go to a desk in the hallway of the school away from classroom distractions so that they can concentrate better.

The automatic repetition of a response is called "perseveration." It is another of the behavioral characteristics of the brain-injured child. Perseveration appears as the repetition of an act, or a response, after the need for the act or the response has passed. The act is continued after it ceases to have meaning or purpose. The response is perpetuated after the situation which first elicited it has passed. The perseveration of an activity or response causes the child to engage in meaningless repetition, like a phonograph needle which becomes stuck in the groove of a broken record and plays the same phrase over and over again. Sometimes, the brain-injured child sounds like a broken record when he repeats the same words or phrases again and again. The term, perseveration, suggests perseverance. But while the latter involves the conscious structure of a goal and indicates purpose, the former is both goal-less and purposeless.

The normal child may repeat acts or words and phrases, but in subtly different ways and in different contexts. He derives satisfaction from the repetition. There is little indication that the brain-injured child derives any satisfaction from perseverative activity. It is thought that perseveration is a form of involuntary and automatic behavior. It frequently appears to take the place of voluntary and goal-directed activity. It fills in a gap for which the child has no appropriate response and usually indicates that the child has failed to perceive accurately the structure and meaning of the new situation. In situations in which the brain-injured child is required to select a response, he may give a per-severative response instead, that is, a response which is only remotely or even not at all related to the stimulus situation. The response is one which was appropriate in another context and which was approved as "right."

A child may also perseverate behavior patterns. At age seven, J. misplaced his coat at school. After school, he could not find it. His teacher and later his parents joined in a search for the coat. It had vanished. After an intensive search was acted out, punctu-ated by scoldings and recrimination, the coat had to be abandoned. The next day it turned up in a classmate's locker. For more than a year afterward, J. hesitated to take off his coat in school or in any place where he felt unfamiliar or insecure. When he was persuaded to remove it, he became anxious and wanted to run back repeatedly to the cloakroom to see if it was there. His explanation was that his parents wanted him to take care of his own things.

In the coat episode, the child's behavior appeared to be neurotic. The fear of again losing the coat and disappointing his parents had become perseverative. J. kept playing back the anxiety and guilt which had been dinned into him at the time of the incident.

The child may perseverate emotional experiences as well as the details of learning and social situations. Like the needle stuck in the groove, he plays back the same response over and over again. Generally, the child is not able to break off a perseverative activity after the initial stimulus has passed unless he is distracted by another stimulus or unless his attention is called to the repetition. Children who perseverate are usually not aware of the repetition. However, older children recognize the error or repetitive response as occurring "in spite of" themselves. In school a child may remark "I don't know what's the matter, but I keep making the same mistake over and over."

Like other physiologically based behavior of the brain-injured child, perseveration is a handicapping activity. It substitutes an unproductive expenditure of energy for a productive one. The child tends not to be aware of the difference. In learning, perseveration may be a serious drawback. It slows down the child's progress. Once he has made an error, that is, once he has organized the stimulus in a given way, it is difficult to change the patterning of his original erroneous percept and he will tend to perpetuate the error.

Perseveration is not exclusively a characteristic of brain injury. It may appear in the young normal child, but to a lesser degree. Many of the behavior anomalies of the Other Child are also seen in young normal children, but rarely in so exaggerated and persistent a form. Under emotional stress, even adults may perseverate or demonstrate disinhibited behavior. These are symptoms of disorganization and disorientation which may only be momentary for the normal person under stress but which are chronic for the brain-injured child—less so when he is not under stress and more so when he is.

Because of his difficulty in organizing, the brain-injured child does not meet new situations with ease. He may become excited with the sudden wealth of new stimuli and disinhibitedly run from one to another, touching and asking about them, to the annoyance of his parents. He has not developed the ability to sit in one place and organize his environment with his eyes.

Another brain-injured child may seem timid or even afraid of new situations. Experience has taught him that organizing, or structuring, a new environment is difficult and that he will feel uneasy or distressed until he has been able to make some meaningful order out of the jumble of separate parts. In some instances his behavior in situations he cannot structure may even resemble panic.

Eight year old R. passed a yard in which a dog began barking at him behind a fence. Terrified, R., who had a dog of his own and was not afraid of dogs, ran away screaming. R.'s flight seemed ludicrous to his playmates who were aware that the dog could not reach them because of the fence. Even after R. was made aware of this, he would repeat his flight whenever the dog barked at him. Not only was his response inappropriate for his age in the first place (because the circumstances did not give him time to perceive the structure of the situation) but he repeated or perseverated it long after he had correctly organized the relationship of the dog, the fence and himself.

In order to protect himself from the disorganizing effect of environmental changes the brain-injured child may become a strict adherent of fixed routines. He will seem inflexible. If he is accustomed to a certain furniture arrangement, he will object to any changes. If he walks to school by a certain route he may protest going another way. If he knows a certain classroom routine he will be acutely distressed if it is not followed. Routine which limits the number of new situations that must be organized is growth-promoting in the life of the young brain-injured child just as is the exclusion of unnecessary distractions. It is equally important, however, to introduce deviations in the routine and the necessity for organizing new situations as soon as the child has developed the perceptual skill which is required to handle them.

For reasons not yet fully understood, the brain-injured child's emotional tolerance is low. Since his grasp of reality tends to be incomplete, a sudden shift in his routine may upset him, toppling a structure he has organized only with difficulty. It might be speculated that this child is subject to an endless conflict with chaos during most of his waking hours, and that this takes its toll of him. We do observe that the Other Child sometimes suffers an inward, emotional collapse, or what may appear to be such a collapse. Suddenly, for no observable reason, he may interrupt an activity and begin weeping. This breakdown may appear to have no connection whatever with what he happens to be doing at the moment. It usually follows a period of sustained effort to mobilize his faculties in the performance of a task. The breakdown may come after he has successfully completed the task. This behavior we call a "catastrophic reaction." The child appears to react as to some great catastrophe, although outwardly nothing significant has happened to him.

These breakdowns may sometimes resemble temper tantrums. The child seems to go to pieces. But there is no temper in the catastrophic reaction of the brain-injured child. It is not a tantrum, but a collapse that he exhibits. It is a compound of frustration and anger and a yielding in helplessness and inner anguish, to an overwhelming demand. One frequently hears parents of brain-injured children describe how it happens. The story usually begins with, "For no reason at all, he just burst out crying...."

Characteristically, a catastrophic reaction does not last long. It passes as quickly as it comes. When it is over, it is usually all finished. The child is then as he was. He may resume an activity, preferably something other than the one in which he was engaged at the onset of the reaction.

How do parents cope with catastrophic reaction? When the child suffers such a collapse, they may help him by comforting him, talking to him quietly and reassuringly until he has regained his composure and then steering him into another activity.

One of the most baffling reactions of the brain-injured child is the behavioral "explosion." It is a sudden, violent eruption of physical activity. The child may suddenly loose a wild shriek, start running about or jumping up and down, stamp his feet, wave his arms, strike out at another child, push someone, kick or throw a toy across the room.

Many reports of brain-injured children include such complaints as "suddenly, out of the blue, he . . ." did thus and so. Why? The behavior becomes more strange when the answer is sought in terms of "what happened to him?" Usually nothing happened to him, nothing that normally would account for such behavior. Yet, some stimulus opened the floodgates of accumulated energy and released it without warning. How does this occur?

To some observers, the explosion appears analogous to the breaking of a dam, with the quick, uncontrolled release of stored energy. In the light of recent behavioral studies, the analogy seems to have validity. It is suggested by these studies that inborn patterns of movement, like the suckling reflex of the infant, exist in human beings as in animals. Such innate movement patterns, sometimes thought of as "instinctive" appear to be "built in" as a function of the nervous system.

These movements are triggered by certain stimuli which act directly on a mechanism which releases energy specific to the movements. The mechanism seems to operate with discrimination, in the way automatic doors of a supermarket swing open when the beam affecting a photoelectric cell is broken. When the release is tripped, energy flows to power a specific set of muscular activities.

It is further supposed that a reservoir of energy is built up in the organism to power these specific activities. This "action-specific energy," as it is called, may accumulate like water piling up behind a dam. The greater the accumulation, the weaker the stimulus required to break the dam—and the more violent becomes the overflow.

Infants commonly exhibit explosive behavior. In the infant, such behavior is expected and acceptable. The infant after a period of quiet may suddenly kick his feet, wave his arms, babble, coo or gurgle seemingly with all his might. As the infant develops, however, much of the accumulated action-specific energy is drained off by the increasing number of responses he is able to make to his environment. In the normal child, this energy tends to be released as it is built up, so that it is not only more controllable but also less violent. The child may be able to control it until a situation arises when he knows it is acceptable to release it. It may appear as the child's "normal exuberance" when he emerges from school with a rush and a shout.

In the brain-injured child, however, action-specific energy may not be drained off as steadily as in the normal child, because the former does not make as many perceptual and conceptual responses as the latter and is also less able to use up his energy in purposive motor activity.

Because of the paucity of his mental activities, the brain-injured child, if he is in a situation requiring restraint and inhibition, tends to accumulate action-specific energy to a greater degree than the normal child. As the energy level rises, the strength of the stimulus required to release it becomes less. Thus, a stimulus pattern which would not affect the normal child may trigger the sudden release of stored up action-specific energy in the brain-injured child. Stimuli which are tolerated adaptively in the forenoon of a school day may not be successfully handled in the afternoon. Unable to control the intensity of his response because of the energy accumulation, the child just "lets go."

Sometimes, the explosion follows frustration. A child unable to untie a knot in his shoe pulls it off and hurls it across the room. Or he may throw a toy against the wall if he finds he cannot make it work. Mingled in his reaction is a strong desire to complete the activity, the blocking of his first attempt at solution, a perceptual and conceptual poverty which does not suggest other solutions, disgust with himself and the object, and final release of the accumulated energy.

When the child's ability to control exaggerated responses is poor, it is said that his emotional tolerance is low. In group situations, at school or at play, the child is subject to many kinds of excitation. He is likely to overrespond if he is teased, called a name or accidentally jostled.

The persistence of excitability, low frustration tolerance or explosive behavior in the brain-injured child is a formidable behavioral handicap. It will prevent him from adjusting to the normal classroom situation. It may tend to isolate him from neighborhood play groups and activities.

While the brain-injured child may slowly tend to "outgrow" his exaggerated emotional responsiveness as his perceptual and conceptual ability increases with maturity, he tends not to outgrow it soon enough unless he receives special help.

Hyper-response, from our observation, is most effectively reduced first by protecting the child from overstimulation and second by enabling the child, through a program of education, to increase the number of responses he makes in all situations so that the reservoir of action-specific energy is maintained at a controllable level.

As the child improves in perceptual and conceptual activity, he becomes more adept at channeling his energy into acceptable patterns of response. Recently, some of the tranquilizing drugs have seemed to be effective in reducing the frequency and intensity of the excessive emotional discharge. But this is a temporary and not always satisfactory solution.

In this discussion of behavior, we have been concerned only with those aspects particular to brain-injured children. Many other behavior disorders may be observed in the Other Child as in normal children. We have sought to point up those which appear to be results of the child's condition in order to emphasize the involuntary nature of some of his behavior which may appear willful—but over which he has little control.

Additionally, a great deal of the child's faulty response to social situations may appear to be misbehavior when it is more nearly miscalculation. In games with other children, the brain-injured child may be disruptive because he fails to perceive the structure of the game and therefore cannot comply with what is expected of him. It is said he cannot "get along" with other children. He cannot frequently because he does not know how.

In many cases, the disability of the brain-injured child is revealed most conspicuously in his behavior. He may not be visibly crippled. His appearance may be perfectly normal. It is mainly in his behavior, through the responses that are otherwise than normal, that he demonstrates his invisible crippledness.

CHAPTER VI

MANAGEMENT: The Other Child at Home

The basis for the successful management of the brain-injured child whose behavior is otherwise than normal is an understanding of his "otherness." This quality of "otherness" generally is expressed in a failure to conform to expected modes of conduct in his age group and milieu. It appears in frequently recurring forms of behavior such as hyperactivity, perseveration, inflexibility, distractibility, irritability, disinhibition and the tantrumlike catastrophic reaction.

Many brain-injured children begin to show behavior difficulties at the age of three or four. While some of these difficulties are similar to those displayed by nonbrain-injured children, they may differ in frequency, intensity and persistence. Indeed, much of the behavior difficulty of the brain-injured child at an early age seems to be an exaggeration or extension of that displayed by the nonbrain-injured child.

The normal child is active; the brain-injured child, hyper-active. The normal child is disinhibited on occasions; the brain-injured child is more so on more occasions. The normal child sometimes has tantrums; the brain-injured child has tantrums for trivial reasons.

The similarities in behavior disturbances between the younger brain-injured and nonbrain-injured children tend to confuse and delay recognition by the parents of the child's problems. At age three or four, the brain-injured child may be regarded simply as a "difficult" child.

His difficulties tend to increase as he grows older and more is expected of him. In socialization with other children, he seems to have a great deal of trouble. Although he wants to, he does not get along with them. Parents notice he is frequently excluded from a play group or active only on the periphery. He is set upon and driven away by the others more and more often until rejection becomes a pattern in his relations with playmates.

On their part, the parents become more and more uneasy and protective toward the child. Sometimes, it may seem to them that he must constantly be defended against others. Within the household, the child's frequent outbursts, his apparent lack of co-operation and his periods of negativeness become incomprehensible and disruptive. Outside the household, he may be viewed as a "badly spoiled" or "willful" child.

In acting out his problems, the brain-injured child projects his dilemma to the parents. Until they come to an understanding of the basis of the child's difficulties, they are powerless to help him or to help themselves.

Every child who displays behavior problems is certainly not brain-injured. Not every brain-injured child has behavior disturbances. But most of the brain-injured children of normal or near normal intelligence whom we have seen exhibit some of these disturbances. And it has been our experience that the behavior disturbances of the brain-injured child can be relieved most effectively by a program of management which takes his handicap into account.

Using this approach to the problem of managing the brain-injured child, we can describe methods of handling him which may help him establish better relationships within the family and outside it. These methods are oriented to the basic idea that much of the child's behavior disturbance is a consequence of a handicap and that, therefore, much of it can be reduced by helping him overcome the handicap. This means that the handicap must be understood and accepted by the parents as a condition affecting the behavior of the child. And before we describe particular methods of handling the Other Child, we should consider the principles behind them.

First, we believe it is important for the parents of a brain-injured child to realize that while many brain-injured children show similar behavior patterns, there is no behavior "type." Each brain-injured child behaves differently from every other brain-injured child. His behavior, like that of the normal child, is formed by the social group, and the family, in which he lives. He adopts their behavior patterns and internalizes their values. However, all brain-injured children, because of the organic disruption in their mental functioning, tend to behave differently from normal children.

In dealing with their normal children, parents often obtain a great deal of assistance from standard guides written for this purpose. To the extent that their brain-injured child conforms to the norm, the recommendations for normal children will help him too. But the further he departs from the norm, that is, the greater his eccentricity, the less appropriate will the standard formulas be.

It follows, too, that traditional ways of rearing children passed on from one generation in the family to the next may be inadequate for the brain-injured child. A mother, training her children, tends to use methods recalled from her own childhood or suggested by her mother as effective, unless she has rejected these methods as unacceptable to her. Here again, with the brain-injured child the time-honored methods may not produce the expected results. The normal child somehow manages to surmount the mistakes made in his upbringing. He develops defenses which help him to pattern a way of life which is more or less satisfactory to him and in harmony with his social group. The brain-injured child lacks the resources and the plasticity to accomplish this without help.

The parents of the brain-injured child, therefore, cannot rely on conventional patterns of child rearing in bringing up their child. The fact that they cannot follow such guides indicates that they must seek other guidance—expert guidance. For the brain-injured child requires a program of management shaped to fit him, and in many respects the program is not conventional.

In the last analysis, however, it is the parents themselves who must develop the child's program. We can only suggest techniques which have helped other children and we can outline the general principles which will aid in planning. It is up to the parents to observe, seek the reasons for the behavior, make the environmental manipulations (including the necessary changes in their own attitudes) and evaluate their effectiveness. Our experience is that when the child senses the parents' efforts to understand him (even if they fall short of perfection) and experiences the relief he obtains from his changed environment, his behavior changes dramatically.

In the Other Child, aberrant behavior is often the first and most dramatic clue to the existence of brain injury. Along with learning difficulties disproportionate to the child's over-all ability, such behavior may be the only visible symptom of his condition.

Brain-injured children who have no motor (muscular) disabilities may appear to be perfectly normal, happy, healthy infants. They may have some difficulty in establishing feeding and sleeping habits but these are "outgrown." They may walk and talk a bit later than normal children or even at about the same time.

Damage to perceptual and conceptual processes may show up in such children only when they reach the ages of three, four or five, when limited play interests and aberrant social behavior become evident. In some children, damage may be so slight that it is not clearly detectable before the age of seven or eight when reasoning and other forms of conceptual thinking are expected in the normal child or when school achievement begins to lag. The child who has suffered brain damage in perceptual and conceptual areas, however, usually displays behavior difficulties soon after he enters the arena of social relationships.

At first, the parents may try to explain away the child's unusual behavior, or ignore it. But they cannot ignore it for long. In nursery school, kindergarten or the first grade of elementary school, the child's deviation may become so disturbing that he cannot be tolerated in these situations. Expulsion of the child from such formalized groups frequently is the first major crisis the family experiences. As the parents look back, they believe they had seen it coming. Somehow, they had hoped he would "straighten out." But this child cannot "straighten out" unless he has help.

In many instances, the child's behavior difficulties become so acute that he becomes severely disruptive in the life of the family. A second crisis has appeared. If the parents have not acted before, they must act now. What can they do? Out of their bewilderment there sometimes arises a sense of guilt. In searching for a reason for the child's otherness, the parents may turn on themselves the "blame" for his condition. Yet, they know, inwardly, that the question of "blame" has no relevance to the problem. Feelings of guilt accomplish nothing except to interfere with an objective analysis of the child's condition.

Nevertheless, many parents have told us of their feelings of inadequacy in dealing with the child. The mother, especially, tends to feel inadequate, for society places the responsibility of managing the child principally on her. She cannot manage this child. Consequently, she may reason, she cannot manage any child.

Feelings of guilt and inadequacy are some of the detours parents must learn to avoid in dealing with the management problem. When such feelings exist in the parents they are inevitably transmitted to the child, feeding his own feelings of insecurity and anxiety as he grows up in a world which to him appears insecure, confused or even hostile.

The accidental nature of brain injury leaves no room for guilt. But it is no wonder that parents may feel inadequate. The brain-injured child presents a highly complex and specialized problem. It is usually entirely outside the experience of the parents and the family group.

The big step the parents find they must take in dealing with the child's problem is to secure competent, professional help. A diagnosis should be sought in which the child's condition is clearly defined and explained. If the diagnosis indicates that the child has suffered brain damage, an assessment should be made of the child's potential. A psychologist can determine in a general way what can be expected of the child under certain conditions of optimum management and to what extent the child can be educated.

There are minimum requirements the child must meet if he is to be considered a subject for education and rehabilitation by methods presently known to us. If he does not meet these standards, our present efforts are not effective in rehabilitating him. In that case, only partial rehabilitation can be accomplished and the expert can recommend whether this can best be done at home or in the protecting environment of an institution.

If it is concluded that the child should have institutional care the question the parents must decide is whether it is required immediately or whether it can be postponed. If the child is so severely damaged that his care is burdensome to the parents and his presence inimical to the welfare of other children in the household, then he should not remain at home. However, if the child can remain in the home, it may be advisable for him to remain as long as possible.

Ultimately, the decision to place the child away from home is up to the parents. Where institutionalization is necessary to protect the child, we feel that training in his own home will help him acquire social habits which will make institutional adjustment easier for him.

Let us suppose the child is on the borderline between educability and institutional care or between mental retardation and normalcy. The question then becomes how much of a financial investment can be made in his rehabilitation against the probability of results. This is not as calculating a proposition as it may seem. Parents should be aware that formal training for the brain-injured child may be expensive. It may involve financial sacrifices that could affect other children in the family adversely. On the other hand, it may be an investment as important to the child and the family as a college education to his brothers and sisters. Again, this is a question which only the parents can decide. In a situation so highly charged with emotion, it may be difficult for the parents to make a decision in a reasoned way, yet a rational course is critically important for the whole family.

These are some of the facets of the management problem at the outset. It is only after they are faced that the problem can be dealt with in an effective way. The brain-injured child who does not appear to meet the requirements for effective help we can give him, or who is borderline in this respect, appears frequently. However, we find a large number of brain-injured children who can be helped to become well-adjusted and self-sufficient individuals.

When this assessment is made by the expert or suggested as a possibility, the path of the parents is clear. They must learn how to manage the child and arrange for an adequate educational program. Educating the Other Child will be discussed in another chapter. The initial problem is managing him. And in this, the attitudes of the parents toward the problem become extremely important.

The brain-injured child presents a unique challenge to his parents. Although he has suffered damage to the same organ as the cerebral palsied child, he usually does not receive the community sympathy and understanding extended to the cerebral palsied child. And special facilities for educating the Other Child in public school systems are rare indeed.

Since the Other Child's difficulties are often most obvious in behavior, he and his parents frequently encounter antipathy, rather than sympathy, in the community. Otherness in behavior is usually a mystery to the community, especially in those where the cultural emphasis is on conformity and ability to compete and cooperate.

If the child resides in a densely populated district of multi-family dwellings, in which play patterns are rigid and restrictions myriad, he faces more difficulty than if he resides in a neighborhood of single homes or in the country. Residence thus becomes a factor in the management of the child.

Brain injury of the type we have been describing is not widely understood as the cause of many behavior aberrations. Consequently, the community may tend to regard these aberrations as willful or the result of parental failings rather than as visible evidence of the child's invisible crippledness. Such an attitude in the community, of course, tends to compound the problem of the parents in managing the brain-injured child who has behavior difficulties. In some communities, however, parents of brain-injured children have formed organizations to share their problems, inform the community of the nature of the child's behavior difficulties and enlist community support for educating and rehabilitating brain-injured children.* Where such organizations exist, parents find it easier to mobilize community support and professional help. Otherwise, parents are forced to "go it alone" in their efforts to find a solution to the child's problems.

Organizational support and professional understanding of the brain-injured child's needs help the parents adopt a positive attitude toward the problem. Such an attitude is essential if the child is to be managed successfully at home.

Parents may expect to find that the development of the brain-injured child is different from that of the normal child. The normal child tends to develop in the normal manner in spite of what his parents may do or fail to do for him. Good family relationships are important for the emotional well-being of every child, but even where these relationships are not wholly satisfactory, the normal child tends to develop in an expected manner. This is not the case with the Other Child. Every step in his development may present a crisis which has to be dealt with specifically. Recognized patterns of mental and emotional development are distorted in the growth of the Other Child, so that his development is not predictable in terms of the normal developmental profile.

Parents cannot explain or anticipate the behavior of the brain-injured child by recalling their own behavior at his age or by comparing him with normal brothers or sisters. His development may not be like that of his parents or siblings because his mental functioning is otherwise than normal. Nor can the parents expect him to follow the behavior patterns of the group, since he differs from the group because of disturbances in perceptual and conceptual processes and frequently is unable to comprehend the patterns of group behavior. Thus, parents should be prepared for differences in the Other Child and understand that these differences are the result of his handicap. It is only by

* Two of these organizations are the Fund for Perceptually Handicapped Children, Inc., Evanston, Ill. and the Society for Brain-Injured Children, Inc., Milwaukee, Wis.

teaching and managing the child in terms of his handicap that these differences can be reduced and the child can be helped to respond in a more normal way to his environment.

Society in America is especially conscious of the child. It expects him to partake of the fullness of life in a rich and productive economy. As part of the immigrant heritage, it is expected that the child will rise above his parents on an economic and social scale. When this expectation is applied to the brain-injured child, it may impose a formidable pressure on him, especially when he understands he is a disappointment and a failure in the eyes of his parents. If he is accepted as he is, a seriously handicapped human being, it is more likely he will receive the love and understanding he so desperately needs.

Yet, although he may be permanently handicapped, his potential development should not be disregarded or underestimated. Parents invariably ask: "What kind of an adult will this child become? Will he be able to take care of himself?"

We believe that the brain-injured child who is capable of being educated and who receives an adequate education can become an independent, self-sufficient and well adjusted adult. But this child usually needs special help to achieve his full potential. If he does not receive this help, then he may not develop as adequately as he might if he does receive it.

The basis of his successful adjustment in later life is an adequate adjustment in the family, and the role of the parents in enabling him to make this adjustment is of critical importance.

Managing the Other Child is a full-time job. It is not beyond the ability of parents who work at it, but it is a job that must be learned.

In the rearing of the Other Child, little can be left to chance. The normal child can be expected to equalize through his own resources the defects in his upbringing, but the Other Child lacks this gyroscopic ability.

When the Other Child is one of a large family, one of two plans may be made. Either the mother needs a helper who will take over part of the household routine and leave her free to devote as much time as she needs to this child, or it may be practical for the assistant to take over the supervision of the brain-injured child for short periods of time in order to give the mother time for a much needed rest.

The Other Child should have a room of his own. If he has no place to play but the living room, he cannot be expected to refrain from damaging the furniture. The damage he does is not necessarily destructiveness, but a result of his awkwardness or his failure to comprehend fragility—to understand that a lamp may break if it falls to the floor.

Also, he needs a place of his own where he can play without being disturbed by other persons, especially at times when he wants to retire and be alone. These are usually times of stress. He needs a quiet place to which he can retreat.

He should have a fenced yard. This protects him from the dangers of the street, which he may not recognize as early as normal children do, and enables the mother to regulate the number of children he plays with.

Too many children and too much noise confuse and irritate him. They result in a progressive weakening of controls and stimulate responses which appear to be antisocial. His striking or pushing another child in a play situation may not necessarily be aggression. It may be an expression of his effort to push away from himself the confusion of many children, which he cannot tolerate and which, for him, constitutes unbearable pressure. Or it may represent an effort to approach them through physical contact, but lacking the modulation of the normal child, he strikes or pushes without restraint.

His own room and his own yard are basic necessities for the Other Child. He must have space. It is important to him that the family live in a single house on a roomy lot. Without living space, he succumbs to the overstimulation of the crowded neighborhood and this contributes to his confusion, making him more hyperactive, untractable and emotionally upset.

For the brain-injured child between two and four years old, the multifamily dwelling is not suitable. He cannot stand living in a small apartment as well as the normal child, and he cannot be allowed to play in the street without constant supervision by an adult. The crowding in of persons in a densely populated neighborhood increases friction for the child and makes the relaxing of behavior problems in the home extremely difficult.

The child's immediate residential environment thus becomes an important factor in his management. Congestion should be avoided, whether it is the congestion of the overcrowded flat or of the modern, multifamily dwelling project.

Parents will find that, no less than with the crippled child, the brain-injured child's handicap must be recognized. How often have the parents of a brain-injured child been told by grand-parents or other relatives: "There's nothing wrong with that child; you're just spoiling him." Relatives need to be assured that what may appear to be spoiling is in reality an effort to bring child and environment into harmony.

When the parents understand the child's condition, they must learn to anticipate the responses he tends to make to frequently recurring situations in the household. Those situations which dis-turb him should be altered or eliminated, at least while he is in the house, and until he can cope with them.

For example, long telephone conversations by the mother may be annoying as they interrupt the activities of the household and force the brain-injured child to endure long delays. If this is the case, the mother arranges her telephoning at a time when the Other Child is out of the house or asleep by tactfully telling her friends that she is busy and will call them back later. In many ways, activities in the home must be geared to the brain-injured child's needs since he does not have the ability to adjust easily to situations which disturb him.

The Other Child as a rule enjoys people and may be fond of friends and relatives. They enhance his feeling of family security. But they can become a severe strain on him if they drop in fre-quently during the day when he needs the mother's attention or if they stay long and overstimulate him. Afternoon teas and bridge parties in the home which fill the house with chattering strangers may be extremely difficult for him to cope with. If this is so, he will demonstrate his difficulty by "acting up." Try-ing to discipline him usually increases his tension and anxiety.

In many ways, the parents find it necessary to change house-hold habits when it becomes apparent to them that such habits contribute to the child's confusion or anxiety. If the family does not have a fixed routine, it should adopt one for the sake of the Other Child. If he tends to get up at seven a.m., he should get up at that time every day. If he has breakfast at eight, he should have it at that time every day. If he goes into the yard at nine, then at nine he should go there. If the weather prevents this, then a substitute activity should be arranged for him. If a neighbor drops in for coffee or a chat while the child is being bathed or dressed or fed, it is the neighbor who must wait—not the child. If the telephone rings while the mother is in the midst of performing routine care for the child, the mother should not take the time to hold a long conversation.

In managing the Other Child, one premise must be kept in focus—the Other Child is high-priority business. Attending to his needs and carrying out his routine cannot be postponed by casual distractions. He is a continual emergency. Unless the parents recognize this by reducing the tensions to which he is subject in the household, they cannot help him adjust to family life, the basis of his social orientation.

The parents must learn to foresee the effect of specific events and situations on the child. If the mother knows, for example, that the arrival of unexpected guests upsets the child, she should have a plan of action in mind in case they drop in. It may be simply having someone else in the family care for him or take him out for a while.

The parents eventually learn to recognize situations that dis-turb the child and to perceive the storm signals which indicate that he has reached the limit of his emotional tolerance. Preventing an emotional outburst by removing the child from situations which obviously are disturbing him or by altering the situations helps the child organize himself. The outburst itself is a sign of the child's internal disorganization. It is more of a cry of distress than a cry of anger.

We cannot dwell on the emotional difficulties of the Other Child, except as they relate directly to his handicap in perceiving and conceptualizing situations. Some specific behavior problems in the home, we have found, are not as mystifying as they might first appear if they are regarded in terms of his physiologic difficulties.

The parents of a nine year old brain-injured boy complained that he would become an unmanageable behavior problem when they had guests in the house, especially for dinner. Even when the guests were expected, their mere presence disturbed him so much that the parents considered isolating themselves from all callers. When guests came for dinner, the boy would jump on the chairs, turn out the lights, eat a few bites at the dinner table, run out of the room, throw food on the floor. Ordinarily, the child, while not easy to manage, did not perform in this way. The child's behavior when guests were present seemed to be an exaggerated form of restless uncertainty. The boy's inability to restructure the home situation when guests were present resulted in an immense anxiety. This he acted out with the wildest kind of behavior. He simply could not tolerate the uncertainty which the arrival of dinner guests introduced into his structure of the family routine. The guests seemed to break down the whole pattern of his family living.

Normal children can tolerate some degree of uncertainty. The brain-injured child usually cannot. The normal child understands that the altered behavior of the parents when guests are present is temporary and the child's reduction to a lesser status than customary is temporary.

The arrival of the visitors introduced a new element in the brain-injured child's notion of his habitual relationship with the parents and in the customary routine. He had to remain quiet while the visitors were talking. Their best-intentioned references to him bewildered him and the fact that they were there only temporarily and would not be permanent additions to the household eluded him. He could not tell what they were doing there because the concept of a visit, especially for dinner, could not be reconciled with his structure of the family routine. The child demonstrated this by continually asking the visitors: "Are you going home? When are you going home?"

Superficially, the question sounded rude and the child was rebuked. But he asked it out of anxiety, not rudeness. Consequently, he could not understand the purpose of the rebuke. It meant to him that whenever visitors came, he was rejected; his brightness as a luminary in the family faded; his security was threatened.

On the basis of this analysis of the child's seemingly bizarre behavior when guests came to the house, the parents were advised to help the child structure the guest situation. When guests were expected, the parents would brief the child in advance. They would tell him that guests were coming for dinner; that the visitors would ring the bell at about 6:30 p.m.; that they would be greeted, would remove their coats and hats and hang them up in the hall closet; that cocktails would be served before the dinner and that afterward everyone would go into the dining room where the children would not be expected to take much part in the conversation. After dinner, everyone would go into the living room. The children would say good night and mother would take them up to bed. Some time after that, the guests would leave.

When this was done, the nine year old boy who had been such a problem when dinner guests were present ceased to be a problem in this situation. After the first thorough briefing, he behaved so well that the parents could hardly believe it was the same child. Thereafter, a thorough briefing on the expected arrival of guests never failed to result in the boy's acceptance of such a change with no remnant of his former disturbed behavior.

What the parents had to do in this instance was to help the boy restructure the family situation when guests were present. They did not "correct" the boy's behavior in doing this; they simply eliminated the cause of the misbehavior by dealing specifically with the organic disability which had produced it, that is, the failure to perceive the new pattern. In this way, they expanded the boy's social horizon by enabling him to make an adequate response to the guest situation. They also brought peace and quiet to the household when guests appeared. It was a double victory and an important one for the child. He had learned to fit into a new situation.

The younger brain-injured child might not be handled so successfully with this approach and other techniques might be necessary to enable him to cope with the intrusion of others in his household. But frequently the key to the Other Child's misbehavior can be found in his inability to structure situations, and helping him to structure them as others do may go a long way toward enabling him to behave in an acceptable way.

A little thought will show how this approach can be helpful in other situations. For example, a brain-injured boy broke his arm on the playground during recess. His reaction was acute panic. The teacher explained to him that he would be taken to the hospital where the doctors would set his arm and put it in a cast so that it would heal. She described how this would occur in the most minute detail she could think of. The boy's anxiety subsided and at the hospital his co-operative behavior was praised by everyone who attended him. His panic was only partly caused by the pain and the immediate concern of everyone around him. In large part, it was due to his inability to anticipate or to construct mentally the pattern of events which would follow.

A birthday party is frequently a great strain on a brain-injured child. In making her plans, the mother should keep the festivitives as simple as possible, and the child guests few in number. The activities and the order of their occurrence should be well planned in advance and the possibilities of delays and disturbances (such as insufficiently thawed ice cream) anticipated and avoided. Then the child should be familiarized with the decorated table, the refreshments and any other novel arrangements which have been made. Finally, the events and program of the party should be carefully explained to him beforehand. He is told that he greets the guests at the door, and that he does not open the presents immediately or all at once. Preparing him by describing to him the probable sequence of events will enable him to cope with what is often a kaleidoscopic series of changes from one pattern to another.

In training the brain-injured child to live comfortably within the family, the mother learns to recognize certain times of stress for the child. These are the times when he gets up in the morning, mealtimes, and when he goes to bed at night. Each of these times represents a division of great consequence to the child in the pattern of his day. The easier it is made for him to structure these divisions, the less strain is imposed on him.

The child rises in the morning to face a new round of uncertainties. If he has learned to dress himself, the first uncertainty is: Where are his clothes? These should be laid out for him the night before, even if his mother dresses him, so that dressing does not involve the uncertainty of hunting for shoes or shirts. Sometimes it is advisable to let him participate the night before, at bedtime, in the selection of what he will wear the next day and place the chosen clothes in a given place for the morning.

The washing and toileting of the child should follow the same routine every day. The more routinized this is, the easier it becomes for the child to wash and toilet himself.

In dressing, many brain-injured children have trouble with undershirts and shirts or dresses. The difficulty stems from two sources: the child's physical clumsiness in handling the garment and his problems in perceiving the pattern of its structure with respect to front and back, and armholes and neck openings. A useful technique is to teach the child to look for the label at the collar as a clue to the back, then to turn the shirt, label down, on the bed, and without picking it up again, "crawl" into it.

Teaching the child to button can be done by having him practice on a garment such as a coat with large button holes and big buttons. Teaching him to tie his shoes should be done in stages: first the crossing of the laces is learned, then the knot, and perhaps quite a long time later the actual bow. When the child begins the mastery of tying his own shoes, very long laces, long enough to enable him to make a generous bow that does not slip out of his grasp are useful.

Socks should be loose enough for him to slip on easily. If the child wears jeans, the belt may be inserted in the loops the night before. Some children find this the most difficult thing to do in dressing.

We have found that parents can reduce behavior difficulties considerably by adhering to a schedule which takes into account the child's need for a routine and the times of the day that are critical for him. In the family unaccustomed to any routine, this may appear to be a highly regimented mode of living. The Other

Child is one, we find, who requires orderliness and regularity to fix his habits and to ease the recurring crises he faces during the day. Any program which reduces these crises and smooths the problem of living for him helps him by lessening his tension and provides the preparation for independence and adaptability at a later age.

If the family sits down to breakfast at the same time every morning, it may be desirable for the Other Child to eat with the family, and, as long as he is young, he should be served first. If younger children disturb him, they may be fed separately. It is usually better for the Other Child to eat with his parents, although some brain-injured children prefer to eat breakfast alone and will rise before anyone else and prepare breakfast for themselves when they have learned to do so in order to eat a peaceful, solitary meal. It is important that, in addition to breakfast, other mealtimes be regular for the Other Child, even if they are not regular for other members of the family and he has to be fed separately.

The brain-injured child sometimes develops food idiosyncrasies or rigid patterns of rejection of certain foods which he retains for years. Often the brain-injured child has difficulty in swallowing because of an easily stimulated gag-reflex; or, diminished tongue mobility makes the chewing of certain foods difficult. It is quite common that the rejection of a particular food which had its origin in an organic disability persists as a fixed idea long after the maturation of the organism has corrected the physiologic problem.

It is not infrequent that the child refuses foods which have been associated with some unpleasant experience such as throwing up, or becoming ill, insisting perseveratively that he cannot eat them. He can be shown the error in his thinking by being led in a casual and matter of fact way to accept a small amount of the food in question.

Occasionally he may insist on having a given food for meal after meal. We have known brain-injured children who refused to eat almost everything except milk and peanut butter sandwiches. Such a food perseveration can be broken by withholding the food he insists on until he has learned to eat even as little as a bite of the other foods being served. When he accepts small amounts of a variety of foods, the food on which he had become fixed may reappear on the table.

Because of his tendency to perseverate, and to avoid new experiences, the Other Child tends to fall readily into habitual responses. Once formed, his eating habits are likely to stay with him.

Lest every expression of like or dislike by a child be construed as perseveration, it should be emphasized that the brain-injured child is subject to the fads and antipathies of any normal child in eating. And, like the normal child, he adopts the attitude of one or both of his parents toward food and reflects their conservatism or willingness to experiment.

In eating, the brain-injured child does better if he experiences a sense of accomplishment in cleaning his plate and should be given such small portions that he can do this easily. In getting the food on his fork he is again handicapped by his motor clumsiness and his perceptual problems. He lacks the wrist and finger dexterity to manipulate the fork so that it probes and picks up efficiently with the result that he tends to push the food ahead of his fork rather than getting the fork under it. Perceptually, he does not see how he might help himself by pushing against a larger portion of food or gathering it all together into the center of his plate. We have found that giving a child a utensil called a "pusher" (a small plastic device shaped like a hoe) enables him to get the food on his fork more successfully and avoids the use of fingers as "pushers."

Some brain-injured children overeat. As the child grows older, this tendency becomes more pronounced than not eating enough. The overeating may have nothing to do with hunger; the child overeats simply because he cannot stop eating. The overeating may be reduced by limiting the portion on the child's plate and giving only a little bit more when he asks for a second helping. Overeating is usually perseverative. When the child's portions are reduced, he may actually feel relieved, even though he asks for more. The child may not know when he has had enough to eat. He frequently will eat exactly what he is given to eat, and no more or no less.

The child who is highly distractible at the table can be helped to attend to his food if the mother will reduce the number of extraneous objects—silver, dishes, salt and pepper shakers, sugar bowls, creamers, glasses, flower bowls, figurines, and anything else not immediately needed. If the child plays with the silver instead of eating, one simply removes the silver. The utensil he needs can be restored as he needs it.

In table training, as in every other phase of training, the principle is that the child does not learn simply by words, but by experience. When he plays with the silver, the parent is tempted to say, "Don't play with the silver." But this is not enough. The silver should be removed, casually and objectively as something which is in the child's way in the same manner as one removes such objects from a very young child. Having a completely set place and being able to leave the utensils alone until time to use them is less important for a young child than harmony in his relationships with others at the table.

It is preferable that the brain-injured child not have his own plate or silverware as this has a perseverative potential. In one instance a child refused to eat in a restaurant unless he could take his own plate and utensils along with him.

Of all the social activities the child must learn, the easiest to organize is eating. It is better for him to eat with his family as eating alone serves no social purpose. If he is impatient and unable to wait, he can be served first and his food cut up for him so that he can start while others are being served. Later, as an elementary school-age child, he can be expected to wait until others are served before beginning if this is the pattern of the family.

It is important for him to learn proper table manners since these provide a means of enabling him to organize the meal and also help him to adjust to the social situation at the table. Being children of habit, the brain-injured children who learn good manners do not easily abandon them.

In washing, bathing, dressing and eating the Other Child requires more supervision over a longer period of time than does the normal child. The supervision should be relaxed but continuing until these habits are firmly seated. A large part of the supervision should consist of demonstrating and then asking the child to attempt by himself efficient ways of accomplishing these self-help activities. The more consistently the child is supervised and shown how to care for himself, the faster he learns. The Other Child seldom learns to do things for himself when put on his own, until he has learned to perceive and organize his world more efficiently. The more help and supervision he receives, the more quickly he becomes self sufficient.

This may sometimes involve pointing out to the child what might seem to be self evident or obvious. For example, one child of eight was impatiently stirring and splashing his soup in annoyance because it was too hot for him to eat. His teacher quietly demonstrated to him how he could take a little bit on his spoon from the edges and off the top where it cools first, rather than from the bottom of the bowl. The child tried this new technique willingly and commented after he found that it worked, "Oh, you mean that's all you gotta do?" Very often the child makes a great stride forward in accomplishing some activity simply by being shown "what you gotta do."

When his habits are acquired, the brain-injured child is likely to reject further help. He may declaim that he wishes privacy in toileting, washing and dressing or that he can do it alone. When this happens, the parent knows this part of the training has been accomplished. The child will tend to continue these activities in the same pattern in which they were learned.

His own room is important to the Other Child as a place indisputably his, perhaps more so than to the normal child. The room should be decorated with one theme—simplicity. He should be relieved of the perceptual confusion or the effort required for him to sort out foreground-background relationships and the room should be a place of friendly quiet.

This recommendation for simplicity does not mean austerity. The brain-injured child is just as pleased by aesthetic qualities which are apparent to him as his normal brothers and sisters. But the décor should be uncomplicated. He doesn't need Jack and Jill, Little Miss Muffet, endless lines of toy soldiers marching off the wall or a linoleum decorated with fairy tale characters. Walls painted in an attractive color, or a conservative all-over pattern of wallpaper are more appropriate. He likes a few well chosen pictures or a pin-up board for items of special interest to him. Color appeals to him and is not distracting; it can be artfully used in bedspread, rug, cushions or chair cover.

The arrangement of furniture should be such that it is easy for the child to find toys or clothing. There are reasons for this. At an early age it is distressing to the child to be unable to find what he wants. Later, the parents will want him to assume the responsibility of keeping his room orderly.

One of the best investments for his room is a toy chest or a large wooden box with a lid on it. This permits toys which do not interest him to be kept out of sight and, again, provides the basic pattern for learning orderliness. For the child who can play only a short while with a toy before losing interest in it it is better not to have the toy chest in his room.

A habit should be made of clearing away the toys at bedtime except for a favorite one or two which the child wishes to take to bed with him or leave in view. This procedure establishes for the child the mental set that bedtime is different from playtime. It also arranges the environment so that in the morning when he awakens it is to an orderly room with his clothing—the first task of the day—easily available to him without distractions.

It may seem that the kind of living program we are describing removes all "interesting" stimuli from the child's environment and is therefore the opposite of what is presumed to be good for children. But what is felt to be appropriate for the normal child does not necessarily apply to the brain-injured child.

The goal of the parents should not be to remove all stimulation but to provide controlled stimulation according to the tolerance of their particular child. This will depend on the extent of the damage he has sustained as well as on his age and general maturity. It should change as the child grows and improves in his mastery over his environment.

Persistent supervision until habits are firmly fixed does not make the child helpless or dependent. But again, the supervision should be adequate to the child's age and developmental level and should provide not only for independence in actual execution of the activity but for independence in initiating it and re-membering the sequences involved.

Routine is the cornerstone of the new edifice of behavior which must be built for the child. Its virtue lies only in the possibility it affords of clearly patterning the day's activities, and in helping the child to relegate to an automatic level many activities on which he otherwise would need to expend conscious effort and attention. It makes life easier for him, and consequently more pleasant. This is reflected in his disposition as well as in that of his parents.

Through routine he finds that he can cope with the ordinary details of everyday living without struggling with each and every one. He is then free to meet new situations and learn how to cope with them. To these he will tend to respond with the habits he has learned through his regular routine. If, for example, he visits another home and is required to wash up for dinner, the established routine of washing will enable him to perform more adequately in the strange bathroom, where soap and towels are not in the places he is accustomed to find them at home. His table manners having been fixed by habit will not break down because of the distractions of the strange household.

Routine and habit-fixing reduce the number of stimulus situations he needs to adjust to. The more habitual these daily routines become the less he tends to respond inadequately to similar situations in which the response has not been learned.

The Other Child makes as many demands as the normal child. But the fact of his brain injury does not give him any special license in this respect. Parents should not give in to his whims any more than they would to his normal brothers and sisters. They should avoid the mistake of offering pity (which keeps him dependent and unsure of his own abilities) in place of a constructive and optimistic program planned to further his development.

Providing an appropriate climate for the brain-injured child, however, does not mean that he should be expected to be the equal of a normal child of his age or even intelligence. It does mean seeing him as clearly as possible as an individual with

certain abilities and deficiencies both of which must be understood. It means expecting him to assume the obligations and responsibilities which are required in family living within the limits
of his particular competence. This does mean taking into account
and "catering" to his aberrant mental processes but it does not
mean excusing him from adjusting on account of them.

In the case of the normal child, giving in to his whims and
demands may "spoil" him; in the case of the Other Child it contributes to his deviation.

Doing everything he wants to when he wants to do it makes
him increasingly restless and hyperactive. The child needs to
know that there are limits and that he is expected to observe
them. Lacking controls himself, and lacking the ability to perceive for himself where the limits of a situation might be, he is
made insecure and anxious if they are not clear to him. The
brain-injured child needs to know that there are consistent de-
pendable limits to his own and others' activity and that the
adults on whom he must necessarily depend are able and willing
to insist they be observed.

One of the brain-injured child's difficulties is an inability to
select. When we make a selection, we compare. This process
involves the perception of a number of different qualities in the
objects or activities under comparison, and the anticipation of
the outcome of the selection in terms of lasting pleasure, shared
pleasures, and so on.

Many of the daily activities of the brain-injured child involve
making such comparisons and choosing satisfactorily after the
comparison has been made. Because of his perceptual difficulties
and his problems in thinking ahead the brain-injured child is
confused by too many choices. He finds it difficult to make a
choice, and then, having finally made one, may be unhappy
with it because he perceives later an advantage he overlooked
in the discarded alternative.

The Other Child should be given choices to make, but as a
young child these should be rather easily accomplished and
should not carry great consequences if he selects in one direction or the other. It is preferable to give him a choice between

two possibilities rather than a choice among many. If the children are being given a treat, he should have the choice of accepting or refusing it or of choosing between ice cream and a popsicle. In selecting his clothes he should be given the choice between the striped shirt or the plain one, the blue or the red, but should not be permitted to insist on anything from his closet regardless of its appropriateness to the occasion, the season or his parents' purse.

As the child grows older he should be given reasons for choices which his parents impose and should be helped to share in the thinking which led to the choice. For example, he should learn that certain clothes are for play because they are less expensive than "good" clothes. Many brain-injured children find it difficult to reconcile such discrepancies as the calendar date, and the beginning of the various seasons, with the actual weather. Because it is March 21 and Spring begins officially, the child will want to take out his lightweight clothing despite the fact that in northern latitudes there will still be periods of cold weather. Similarly on the first cool Fall morning the child is convinced that winter is arriving and that he needs his flannel shirt. Many of them become greatly interested in the morning weather forecast in order to help them with the problem of anticipating the day's weather and being prepared for what may develop.

The child's difficulty in making choices extends also to his play. A number of toys given to him on occasions like his birthday or Christmas has the effect of disorganizing him. Each of them attracts him equally. He picks up one, and is attracted by another. Variety becomes sameness to him; multiplicity becomes confusion.

It is generally better for him to have a few toys to play with than a large number. Rather than having them all at once some should be put away to be taken out when he has run out of "things to do."

Many brain-injured children become satiated quickly with a toy or game. The normal child, having identified the nature and purpose of the toy, tries it out in several ways to see how it works, and from this he goes on to invent many variations. His perceptual and conceptual abilities lead him to see infinite possibilities for playing with the toy alone and in combination with other materials.

Because of his perceptual disturbance the brain-injured child may fail to see how certain parts of a toy work, how they may be used and how they cannot be used. He tends to focus on the details of the toy, instead of its function as a whole. He may be fascinated by the wheels of his red truck. The wheels go around. The fact that they are part of the truck and enable the whole truck to move evades him. He may not readily think of the truck as a miniature of a real truck, nor relate the use of the toy to what a real truck does—carry loads. The toy may thus be meaningless to him for what it represents, and he is likely to take the wheels off.

Or he may attempt to make the truck go sideways, instead of backwards and forward. When it does not move sideways, rather than recognizing it is because of the construction of the wheels, he becomes frustrated and angry, attempts to force the toy and often breaks it.

Parents have a tendency to buy the kind of toys for a child they imagine they would have liked at his age, or the kind they like at their age. Maybe this is the reason fathers buy complicated electric trains for little tots, and why many parents are disappointed when the toy they have chosen fails to interest the Other Child.

Giving play things to the brain-injured child should be considered a part of the educative process. In this the parent has to use a little imagination. It is obviously of little help to ask the salesperson, "What do you think would be good for a five year old boy?"

One of the things to be considered is the child's perceptual level. The popular "educational" toys are often not suitable for him because they are designed on the premise that the child user enjoys a normal perception of form and space relationships. In order to be used successfully they require exactly that faculty which is often damaged in the brain-injured child.

It is better to buy him a simple sturdy toy which can survive his initial misuse and which will eventually become a part of his play as he learns to use it properly. If he has a truck which he can't break, which is too heavy to roll fast and which does not move too easily, he will learn to play with it. He finds he can't move it sideways. He likes to push it forward or backward. It will take large and heavy loads. When he learns to play with it, he will play with lighter, more fragile toys of the same kind more appropriately. This kind of toy has some educational value for the child in terms of his disability. However, it is still better if the parent takes the time to show the child not only how to use the toy but some of the possibilities that exist in enlarging the conceptual scheme into which it can fit.

Many brain-injured children are described as destructive but this statement alone is insufficient. Destructiveness results from several factors. It may be that the child has failed to perceive the overall possibilities of the toy and begins to take it apart because he is more interested in the details than in the whole. This is a perceptual or conceptual failure rather than destructiveness, and curiosity on the level of awareness which is within the child's ken. Or it may be that a part of the toy sticks or does not move as the child expects or would like it to and he attempts to force it. The toy is not made to withstand such force and breaks. The child did not mean to do it. He simply did not anticipate the events which could occur.

Sometimes, he may become so annoyed with a toy's failure to perform that he may discard it or throw it against the wall. To the observer, this may appear to be sheer destructiveness. To the child it brings relief. Any object which he cannot manipulate as he wants to has no value to him as a toy and he gets rid of it. It is only a frustration. Later, he may go back to the broken toy and play with it again. His wrecking of it may not have been complete. In fact, he did not mean to break it. He just wanted to get it out of the way.

Another aspect of destructiveness is that the motion of the toy such as a small car excites the child's impulse for more and more movement and stimulates hurtling the car from one position to another rather than moving it with restraint. This is accidental rather than deliberate destruction although the effect on the toy is the same, as is the appearance of the action.

A great deal has been said about discipline for children. What about discipline for the brain-injured child? Should he be disciplined? We believe he should. He must be able to live in society, and discipline is a part of his training.

Punishment will yield only negative results if it is applied to "correct" acts which are a result of his disinhibition, impulsivity or inadequacy of response. These are aspects of his crippledness.

If his "naughtiness" is a result of his inability to respond adequately and his "rebelliousness" or "willfulness" a result of his lack of inhibition and confusion, punishment is futile and only contributes further to the child's deviation.

The Other Child's intense desire to be close to another human being can be used as an influence in his discipline. In a situation where the child has become negative and unco-operative, it sometimes helps to induce him to remain quiet for a few moments while the parent talks to him. This should be done in a quiet relaxed fashion, if possible away from the situation in which the unco-operative behavior was expressed and away from an audience of brothers and sisters or other family members. It is often good to show a physical closeness to the child—when he is very young to take him on one's lap, and when he is older to sit beside him. The parent should wait quietly until the child's initial protests have subsided, and then, in a simple, gentle and direct way talk to him about the episode. The purpose of the talk is to obtain the child's co-operation. This the child will usually give unhesitatingly when he understands what is expected of him and when he feels that the parent is in an understanding rather than a punitive mood.

Such unco-operative episodes usually occur when the child must shift from one activity to another, such as leaving his play in order to go to bed. The parent's effort should be directed toward heightening the value of the new activity in one way or another so that the child will be able to accept it as agreeable to him. For example, the mother may explain that it is time to go to bed, that this is the time he always goes to bed, that all children are going to bed, that when he is ready father will read to him, and so on. She does not threaten or scold him. She persuades him to make the transition from what he is doing to bedtime.

Keeping the child quiet for a few moments helps him by calming him. Talking to him quietly helps establish the human relationship he needs. Explaining the situation to him helps structure the new activity. Pointing out its attractive features makes it easier for him to make the choice.

Brain-injured children seldom are rebellious, although they exhibit a reaction which is similar to it. Real rebellion requires a high degree of conceptual activity. It requires a thorough definition of the situation rebelled against and the selection of a preferable alternative. We do not find that many brain-injured children are capable of this kind of rebellion. What may appear to be rebelliousness is more likely to be resistance to a change in status quo, especially at a time when the child is tired and tense. Helping the child to make the change melts the resistance. This is a kind of discipline that recognizes the child's otherness and at the same time enables him to conform to the behavior expected of him.

When the child throws a toy and breaks it, taking away the toy for a while is better than scolding him. As we have indicated, the child may have thrown the toy impulsively or to get rid of it. Removing it eliminates the disturbance the toy has created. It also teaches the child that when he throws or attempts to break his things he loses them. The parent's attitude in all of these interchanges is extremely important, as the goal is to teach the child consequences of his behavior. This can be learned best if the parent is simply the agent through which these consequences occur, rather than a frustrated, disappointed and annoyed participant.

Discipline must be part of the educative process. And to be effective it must be appropriate to the motive behind the misbehavior. Punishing the Other Child so that he will curb his so-called tantrums or forcing him to behave "like other children" is the same thing as punishing a cerebral palsied child because he cannot run like other children. Both children are crippled as a result of damage to the same organ—the brain.

Through discipline, the child gains insight. He learns the consequence of his behavior. This is the most effective way to reduce his deviation and enable him to behave normally. We speak of discipline rather than punishment for the reason that discipline is part of the child's training. It is not punitive. In the younger brain-injured child, punishment serves no constructive purpose. The child must learn what is good behavior before he knows what is misbehavior. Few of his impulsive, antisocial acts are deliberate or premeditated, but as we have emphasized previously, they result from an inadequate perception of the situation.

In the brain-injured child the mechanism which organizes the behavior he exhibits—enabling him to perceive and structure social situations, develop awareness of social attitudes and develop inhibitions—is not operating in the normal way.

We have described the catastrophic reaction in the brain-injured child as a miniature breakdown of controls. This is what many parents mistake for a tantrum. But it is not a tantrum. It is a collapse. The child's crying is not angry, it is agitated. When the Other Child suffers such a reaction, his immediate need is a period of quiet with a sympathetic person, usually his mother, preferably in his own room. There the mother wipes away the tears and calms him. It is important for the child to have her full sympathy and support. In a short time, usually five to ten minutes, the reaction has passed, the child is as he was, and will resume playing as though nothing had happened.

One way of resolving difficult behavior situations with the Other Child is to remove him from the scene. If he is squabbling in a group, he should be taken out of the group. It is not sufficient to tell him to "behave yourself." But he should not be isolated. Long periods of isolation give him the impression that he is being shunted aside, and this is not the purpose of removing him from the scene of misbehavior. The disciplinary purpose is secondary to the necessity for extricating him from a group situation he obviously cannot cope with. The parent can restore him to the situation by reducing the demands of the situation on the child. This helps him learn to cope with it.

Suppose the child is with a group of children digging in the sand at the beach, and he begins to throw sand indiscriminately.

He is removed from the group to reduce the stimulation which has brought on the impulsive throwing of sand. If the other children have been building a castle or some design the Other Child cannot perceive properly, something simpler for him to do is found. Let's dig a hole. A hole is easy to structure for him. And the digging of it drains off the energy he has been using to throw the sand.

A secondary disciplinary result is the demonstration that if he throws sand in a group of children, he cannot remain in the group. It is probable that the throwing was not emotional, there was no target; it was impulsive, a disinhibited act.

Suppose he was throwing at a target—another child "because he threw sand at me." Few parents are able to solve the question of who did what first. It is not important that guilt be established. Removing the Other Child from the group in this case eliminates the conflict. And this is desirable for the Other Child, because conflict widens his incoherence.

Threats are not effective. He may have difficulty understanding what they mean. They tend to negate the child's desire to emulate good behavior for the purpose of being better able to cope with the world about him. Also, he may not understand the reason for the threat.

Promises of reward (if you eat your peas, you can have ice cream) will help only when the child has recognized achievement as a process by which he masters his environment. To give him a reward merely on the basis of a good result, which may be accidental, is meaningless. The child may not see the relation of the reward to the successfully completed activity, hence nothing is accomplished. We do not recommend that parents use reward to stimulate the child to do something correctly. This tends to increase the pressure on him. It is preferable to share with him in the process of the accomplishment and then to praise him. In many instances, the prospect of reward constitutes a distraction. The child no longer wants his peas; he wants the promised ice cream. He cannot eat the peas while the ice cream is in prospect. If any reward is given to the young child, it should not be announced ahead of time, but given immediately after completion of the successful task.

Often the brain-injured child makes requests which appear to the parents to be not only impractical of fulfillment but ridiculous. They are tempted to assume the child is being unreasonable, possibly even with the purpose of annoying them, and to dismiss the request by ridiculing it. Often such a ridiculous request originates from the child's lack of perception of its obvious incongruence. To point out its foolishness only demonstrates to the child his inability to think as well as others do, and reinforces his already present feelings of insufficiency. It is far better to take his request on faith, and seriously answer it with factual information which, even though it seems obvious, the child may not have related to this situation.

A promise to the brain-injured child is a contract. No court can break it. Nor can the parents. No promise should be made unless it can be kept. As far as future events are concerned, it is better to be as indefinite as possible about the whens and wheres of them. It is preferable to postpone announcements of such coming events as a trip to see Grandma or a vacation until the event is close at hand, and then to qualify it heavily. It is better not to say: "We are going to visit Grandma Sunday afternoon." It is better to say (on Friday): "Maybe we will visit Grandma if we can get away on Sunday."

The Other Child does not qualify experiences readily. But he has to learn the "maybes" of experience. Certainty is easy for him to accept. Harder for him to visualize is the alternative. So he has to be told about the alternative of going to visit Grandma which is *not* going to visit Grandma. Then he can accept a cancellation of the trip if it is raining, or the car won't start or Grandma is ill.

For an important change in family routine, the child should be fully prepared. The change should be described to him shortly before it begins. But it can be discussed with him in a general, qualified way before that. He should not be taken by surprise when the family moves from the residence to another or from one city to another. Preparation enables him to understand what is going on.

Verbal communication with the Other Child is an important

part of the management problem. It is useless to give him even a short instruction while his attention is occupied with something else. He may even reply in order to indicate that he has heard and then not have perceived any of the content of the parent's remarks. Or he may be unheeding, giving the impression that he is deliberately not listening. The truth of the matter is that while he has one channel of perception open to stimuli the others are functionally closed.

The most successful approach is to call the child, or even to tap him on the arm to obtain his attention, and lead him a short distance away from the toys or television set, stating that you have something to say to him. Then with his full attention, the instructions may be given simply, directly and briefly. This gives the best assurance that they will be carried out.

Verbal instructions can be given in such a way that they aid the child in the performance of a task or a chore. The choice of language is the key, however, to making the instructions work. Usually, the instructions should be given in sequence: "Here is fifty cents. Go to the store on the corner. Ask the man in the white apron for a box of cocoa. Give him the 50 cents. He will give you change. Put the change in your pocket. And bring the cocoa back." The sequence enables the child to pattern the errand, and he will usually do it well.

Often if the child fails to complete an errand to the parent's satisfaction he will reproach the parent with the remark, "But you didn't tell me to do that." The parent has not been explicit. He has expected the child to fill in—to assume what was unsaid. The brain-injured child does not bridge these gaps easily because of his conceptual difficulties. He is justified in resenting being held to an accomplishment which was beyond his ability.

Many brain-injured children question constantly or persistently remind parents of a promise. The child who reminds excessively may do so for two reasons. First, from his own experience he knows that he himself forgets and that things slip out of his mind. He assumes that others are as he is and reminds them to reassure himself that the awaited event has not been forgotten. Many brain-injured children have a poor concept of the passage of time. The word, "afternoon," does not convey the whole concept of a full morning of play, lunch, a rest and more play before the event is to take place.

Children who question constantly are usually seeking an answer to a point which is confused. Adults are accustomed to give the child categorical instructions such as "Jimmy, don't step on the grass." To the child with conceptual difficulties, such an instruction is manifestly incomplete. He has seen people walk on the grass. He has even done it himself and no one has restrained him. He has been on picnics where much effort has been spent in finding a good patch of grass to sit on. His problem now becomes one of determining whether this instruction means "From now on, don't ever walk on any grass," or "Don't walk on this particular grass but that over there is all right to walk on." He attempts to sort out through his questions the possible situations in which these instructions apply or do not apply. It should be remembered that part of his problem is a desire to conform. How can he if he does not know in what way? Such a child's questions will end if he is given a full explanation of the meaning of the statement, including what grass may be walked on, under which conditions and when.

Brain-injured children of school age often have considerable difficulty in handling money. While they may know the denominations and coins, many such children cannot handle more money than they need for a specific occasion. Also, they have a tendency to lose it. Money in the pocket is a distraction. Consequently, it does not stay in the pocket long. Out it comes for the child to examine or play with. Something else distracts him momentarily, and the money is gone. What did he do with it? He doesn't know. He guessed he lost it. In handling money, the child has an easier time if he has to carry only the amount he needs for a specific purpose, and only for a short time. Giving him an allowance to teach him the value of money does not work as well as giving him specific sums to spend on specific objects. He may tend to lose a week's allowance the first day. He can control 10 cents a day much more easily than 50 cents a week, and the smaller coin is much less of a distraction.

Coins he is given can be increased in size and value as he

becomes accustomed to handling them. Giving the child a dollar bill before he understands its coin components may be risky. The bill is a piece of paper to him. Even though he may know its value, his tendency to treat it with the casualness of a piece of paper may be especially strong unless it is for the purchase of a specific item.

Outside the home, the Other Child's training continues. His tendency to behave on a lower age level may be noticeable in a restaurant or on a picnic. This and other signs of his deviation, such as grimacing or excessive arm and body movements, may embarrass the parents. In a restaurant, some of his hyperactivity and distractability may be reduced if he faces the wall, and he is more at ease if he is not sitting beside a younger child. Another seating arrangement is to place him so that he is beside his mother and facing his father.

Waiting in the restaurant or in any public place for service is hard on the child, and it is to be expected that he may become restless. Many brain-injured children whose distractibility in restaurants is a problem tend to sit quietly in the dining car of a train. It is probable that watching the scenery flow by provides an organizing focus, so that the activity in the dining car can be relegated to background status. In a restaurant, providing a focus for the child may help reduce his restlessness. Some restaurants which cater to children provide a simple puzzle or a card with a sequence of numbers which the child can follow with a pencil to produce a drawing.

Any method that will help the child organize the restaurant situation will reduce his distractibility and thus improve his behavior. Sometimes it helps to point out the purpose of the various items on the table or in the room, or call his attention to the activities of the waitresses. If the child acts up and cannot be quieted, he must be removed for a while. The mother can take him to the bathroom or lounge. Then he can return to the table. Again, it is important to brief him in advance. And if the family eats out often, eating at the same restaurant makes it easier for the child.

Some brain-injured children, in whom motor areas of the brain have been damaged so that grimacing or peculiarities in gait result, may be conspicuous enough to cause comment. The parents cannot avoid or retreat from these situations. The child is quite aware of them. The situation may be exploited by explaining to the child that there are people in the world who are sometimes rude. This may help the child understand that it is not socially acceptable to stare at persons with physical disabilities.

We have observed that the brain-injured child tends to be more egocentric than the normal child, and one reason for this is his inability to win acceptance in a group. We sometimes find him playing on the periphery of a group of children, acting out his notion of the activities the other children are engaged in, but not a part of these activities. He may experience particular difficulty after the age of approximately seven or eight when children's games become team or group activities.

He cannot play many group games or enter into group activities when he does not perceive the pattern of the games. Consequently, he does not conform to them and is usually expelled from the group as a disturbing influence or a liability to the team. If this is habitual, he will not offer to enter into the group's activities, but, wanting companionship, he will hang around, watch for a while, and then act out his version of the activity by himself.

His lone wolf role is not only a result of the group's rejection of him but of his own difficulty in relating to them. What they are doing does not interest him if he does not perceive the nature of the game or if he perceives only parts of it. Even if he does see the pattern, he may not be able to follow it consistently or to the satisfaction of the other children.

In hide-and-go-seek, the Other Child does not hide successfully. He feels compelled to keep peeking from his hiding place to see what is going on. From the hiding place, he is not able to project in his imagination the activities of the others, who either are hiding or searching. In addition, it is difficult for him to maintain a sense of relatedness to the game without visual contact.

The sense of isolation he feels while hiding is not allayed by the realization that this is part of the game structure because he may not perceive the structure in its entirety. For him, the game proceeds in the sequence of his own activity. He is in the group, then he hides, and suddenly, he is alone. What has happened? He peeks to see, and gives himself away.

As a searcher, his inability to visualize the other children hiding and the places where they might hide makes searching a fruitless task. If he is distracted, he quickly abandons the search. In either case, he does not play the game.

School age children tend to have a rigid concept of the rules of games. This is an age when normal children will argue about the rightness or wrongness of game behavior. The brain-injured child either may not understand the rules or be unable to fit them into the pattern of the game. Or, he may observe one rule, but not another. His rule-breaking proclivity results in his ostracism, because "he doesn't play right" or "he doesn't play fair."

Eventually he will conclude he doesn't "want" to play the games the others are playing. Consequently, the brain-injured child will tend to find acceptance as a playmate with younger children who are more casual about the rules of games and less disturbed by infractions and whose social group organization is not as highly developed.

In many of his childhood social experiences, the brain-injured child is constantly made aware of his otherness. Because of perceptual disturbance, one child may put up his hand to ward off a blow if a child ten feet away picks up a stick. He thinks the stick may hit him. He cannot climb successfully or perform many of the agile stunts of other children because of his perceptual and motor handicaps.

Yet, the Other Child can be taught to play games and it is important that he be taught. He can learn to throw and catch a ball. Usually, this has to be initiated by the parent, since other children will not let him take part in their baseball or basketball games. He can be taught to ice skate, roller skate and ride a bicycle. But many brain-injured children do not learn these skills by themselves.

Outside the home, the child's need for social acceptance should be filled as much as possible. One way of enabling him to have supervised group experience as a young child is to enroll him in a nursery school. But it should be a nursery school whose

teachers are willing to attempt to work with the child after his
condition has been explained to them. Most nursery school teachers can adapt (rather readily) the techniques they have learned
in daily dealings with normal children to the young brain-
injured child. As we have shown, the behavior of the brain-
injured child is much like that of a nursery school child in
that he is easily overstimulated, suggestible, hyperactive and
so on.

For the child who shows early signs of becoming a social misfit, we believe the nursery, play school or kindergarten experience is critical. Here is an opportunity for the child to learn the
elements of behaving in a group. In this experience, the child
should not be segregated. He must learn to try to get along in
normal society outside his own home. However, this normal environment should be as benign and understanding as possible.
The importance of explaining the child's difficulties to a nursery
school teacher in advance and having him accepted on this basis
can be illustrated by the following incident.

During recess at one school, the impulsive children ran to the
gate of the yard to watch a horse pulling a wagon through the
alley. Some of them ran into the alley. This of course could not
be permitted. The teacher warned the children that anyone who
disobeyed the rule about running into the alley would forfeit the
next recess. "If I put out one hand or one foot through the gate,
will I miss recess?" asked the brain-injured child. From a normal
child, this would sound impertinent. From the brain-injured
child, it is a reasonable question. He is trying to understand the
limit of what he can do and cannot do. He may not perceive the
intent of the restriction. If the teacher takes this question on
faith, and replies that, no, he cannot even put out one foot or
one hand, she will answer the question and the child will be
satisfied.

Some children are easily overstimulated and a large group
or a complete school day are intolerable. Their behavior becomes
progressively more disorganized as the day progresses, and as
the child fatigues and is no longer able to organize his world.
Such a child will benefit by being in the group situation only
for a short while, possibly for an hour or even 45 minutes while

the group is engaged in activities which will permit his participation as an onlooker or a peripheral member.

Throughout the child's growing up years his group experiences need to be carefully and wisely chosen. Many parents express concern because their brain-injured child has few friends.
It should be remembered that because of his organic problems
the brain-injured child belongs to a minority. The differences resulting from these problems will make it harder for him to form
as many satisfying friendships as the versatile normal child. It is
enough if the brain-injured child can maintain good casual relations with other children in the school and neighborhood and
acquire, in the course of time, a few real friends.

Our approach to managing the Other Child is predicated on
the fact of his physiological disturbance, and on the realization
that this engages him in a perpetual effort to live at peace with
the world around him. The struggle is real, it is never ending
and it tends to negate the carefreeness of childhood. For the
Other Child is seldom carefree. In this sense, he does not have a
happy childhood as he is constantly engaged in an effort to overcome a handicap.

For many Other Children, childhood is an introduction into a
hostile world, indifferent to their real needs, a world which makes
demands on them they cannot meet. These children work hard
to face up to such an environment almost from the day they are
born. It is mainly when the parents understand what problems
the child really encounters that they can begin to give him the
help he so desperately needs.

The techniques described for working with the Other Child
may be useful in some situations. There are no formulas. The
key to managing him successfully lies in the parents and in their
willingness to understand his otherness.

CHAPTER VII

EDUCATION: The Child at School

Education is probably the most significant life experience of the child in twentieth century American society. Modern life has become so complex that many of its social and economic aspects must be learned in a formal program of education. Education is the way by which much of the culture of today is transmitted to the new generation. Consequently, schooling has become an essential experience in the adaptation of the present-day child to his environment.

This has not always been so. In earlier and simpler cultures, education could be considered a luxury. A frontier society required little formal education for survival, and a primitive society required none beyond the learning of social rites and simple skills.

Even after a minimal twelve years of schooling, no one in our society is well acquainted with the details of the enormous body of technical and theoretical knowledge on which our civilization depends. To become technically proficient in one particular field may require most of a lifetime. Eight years of primary and four years of secondary education are required to establish only the fundamentals which will enable us later to lead independent adult lives.

Thus, in today's world, formal education is a "must" for survival. Illiterates can still get along in some rural regions of this country but even this situation is changing rapidly. In urban centers, literacy is almost a necessity for earning a livelihood and for making an adjustment to city life. Never before in history has education become so critical a factor as it is today. Not only has it become essential for the individual, but it is necessary for national survival.

In recent years, education experts have warned that the teaching of mathematics—the fundamental tool of a mechanical civilization—has become inadequate to meet the increasing demands of a rapidly growing technology. Our expanding population requires constant improvement in the techniques of producing food, housing, clothing, transport and communications.

As new sources of energy are developed to enable the greatest populations in the history of mankind to survive on this crowded planet, the need for technicians, engineers and scientists increases. As a consequence of this relatively recent stress on education the problem of the educationally handicapped child has assumed an importance it has never had in a less complex and less interdependent society. It is partly for this reason that the brain-injured child has become identified as a significant problem in education. A half century ago, such a child could have made, and probably did make, his way in the world, with only the rudiments of educational skills. Today, he would become a public or private charge unless he lived in an isolated farming community.

This is the basic problem posed by the learning difficulties of brain-injured children. It is not simply one of learning for the sake of learning, but of learning in order to exist as a social being.

The importance of education is widely recognized in the constitutions and laws governing education in every state in the union. Each state provides in general terms for the education of all children between the ages of 6 and 18 who can profit from instruction. The education of the physically and mentally handicapped child is assumed to be an obligation of the state and most states have developed programs of special education for the handicapped child. Generally speaking, there are provisions for the physically handicapped and for children with sensory losses in hearing and vision. Some of these programs are elaborate, well planned and ably staffed. There are also provisions for the educable mentally handicapped.

The exceptional child is regarded as a special educational

problem in most states, whether he is physically or mentally handicapped, or whether he is exceptional by reason of extraordinary intelligence and precocity.

How does the brain-injured child fare in this scheme of special education? In our experience, and that of most parents of the Other Child, we are compelled to state he does not fare very well. In a sense, the Other Child is both physically and mentally handicapped. Let us say he is mentally handicapped because he has suffered a physical disability in damage to the brain substance. Further, his physiologic disability has resulted in learning difficulties which are a direct and specific consequence of the brain damage. In this respect, he differs from children who are retarded educationally because of environmental conditions or emotional maladjustment.

Although special education in the nation's public school systems has come a long way in recognizing the requirements of the exceptional child, it has not generally recognized the brain-injured child as a special problem. In most school systems, brain-injured children of borderline or below normal intelligence are not differentiated from retarded children who are not brain-injured. Where this difference is not recognized, the education of the brain-injured child tends to be inadequate in relation to his potential learning ability.

Because their slow progress or actual lack of progress is easily confused with the slow learning rate of the nonbrain-injured retarded child, they are usually classed together in the same program of special education. In general, such programs do not take into account the specific difficulties in perception, language and concept formation of many brain-injured children. As a result, the Other Child often has much the same difficulties in the special class as in the regular classroom. The brain-injured child of normal intelligence may be in the same predicament. He is, rightly enough, classified as "normal" or "average" according to standard intelligence test results, yet he often cannot learn as an average child learns.

Brain injury does not necessarily produce mental retardation although it may diminish intelligence to a level below that which the child might have had without the injury. It does impair the effectiveness with which the child perceives his environment and organizes his perceptions into an accurate model of it. It affects his ability to function, since at various stages of his growth his mental processes are not in step with each other. Some, such as language, may have developed at an average or even above average rate. Others, such as perception, may lag far behind. Because of this discrepancy, the brain-injured child does not enjoy the same advantage as the child whose mental development goes forward on a fairly even front. His mental processes do not play into and support one another as they normally should.

Brain injury may also block the exercise of intelligence by creating a learning handicap. A child with poor visual or auditory recall or a tendency to mishear the sounds or sequence of letters in words will have difficulty in learning to read. This will seriously limit his educational progress and opportunities.

We have found that when a program is developed which takes into account his particular disabilities and helps him to compensate for them, the brain-injured child of normal or near normal intelligence is able to progress in school frequently as well as another child of comparable ability. Conversely, where the school program does not deal with the Other Child's specific learning difficulties, his progress tends to be poor, his performance inadequate and his behavior troublesome.

This conclusion is based on our observations of the progress of children who were enrolled in The Cove Schools, a private school for brain-injured children at Racine, Wisconsin and Evanston, Illinois and in a class in the public school system of Joliet, Illinois which was taught according to methods developed at The Cove Schools. It leads us to a further conclusion: that school systems which make no provision for the education of brain-injured children in terms of their learning disabilities are not adequately discharging their responsibilities in public education.

We believe the education of the brain-injured child begins as early as possible. While it is the responsibility of the state to provide an adequate teaching program for him when he reaches school age, it is the responsibility of the parent to prepare him as fully as possible for the public school. However, the parent should remember that the normal child acquires skills and organizes new experiences easily and that the brain-injured child with perceptual and organizational difficulties does not. The problem of the parent is to provide opportunities for the brain-injured child and to encourage him without pressing him beyond his abilities. The child's interest in and acceptance of the activities which are offered are usually the best guide. A brain-injured child's dislike of an activity or refusal to play is more often than not an indication that some confusion or difficulty exists for him which robs the activity of any element of fun it might have for normal children.

A nursery school for normal children is often advisable if the child's behavior is not too disturbing to the other children. Even if the child can stay for only one hour a day it is valuable. The organized activity with other children of this age helps prepare the brain-injured child for his initial school experience in large part because it gives him normal patterns to follow. Furthermore, it takes him outside the home for a while, relieving the mother of his care during this time. If the child's behavior is so disturbing that he cannot remain in a nursery school, he will benefit from nursery-school type activities given by a tutor. The tutoring should be done by someone other than a member of the family, preferably a teacher, and preferably away from home.

At home, the mother can encourage the child to help in doing simple household tasks. These are an important part of his training and give him a feeling of participation in the household. Such chores help him incorporate processes of orderliness in his experience by showing him what order is.

It is best if the child can be treated, always making allowances for his disabilites, in a manner appropriate for any child of his age. A brain-injured child of nursery or kindergarten age in either chronological or mental development should not be expected to have formal lessons intended to improve his perception. What he does should be fun and in the spirit of play. Wisely chosen activities and materials used with proper encouragement will do the teaching.

For his elementary school years we follow the principle that the child should be encouraged in what he can do well, but not at the expense of what he cannot do well. The Other Child is an organism out of normal balance; we do not wish to accentuate the imbalance. For example, some brain-injured children are highly verbal, but low in performance ability. The low performance is the result of perceptual-motor difficulty, wherein perception is not a reliable guide to the performance of an act. The child perceives and organizes visual stimuli so inadequately that he does not "see" how to put the puzzle together or what he is expected to do in drawing, cutting, pasting, coloring, etc. These children tend to mask their poor performance by substituting talking for doing. The energy normally expended in doing may thus be diverted into talking. If the child is led into doing, his energy will be used in motor activity and less of it will go into verbalization.

Most of us recognize that the tendency to verbalize as a substitute for performance is a rather common characteristic, in which a vicarious feeling of accomplishment is obtained by talking instead of doing. In the brain-injured child whose motor performance is poor, this tendency is heightened. The verbalization not only tends to replace the performance of the task but it tends to interfere with the child's ability to perceive the task as it is. Thus, in verbalizing instead of doing, the child tends to widen his deviation.

In performing a task the child must perceive its structure. The performance itself operates as a feedback and check on the accuracy of the child's perception. In verbalizing, however, the child is not confined to the task structure, nor is there any feedback to inform him whether he has perceived correctly or incorrectly.

One of the reasons brain-injured children impress us as being immature when they reach school age is their lack of perceptual motor development. Hand and eye do not work together in the normal way. The child may place pegs in the holes of a pegboard for a time but it soon becomes apparent that he is not looking at what he is doing. He is looking somewhere else. It appears that he has been placing the pegs by tactual and kinesthetic sensations but he has not organized them into a visual pattern. That is, he has not been "seeing" what he has been doing.

The motor manipulations have been guided almost entirely by his sense of touch, while his visual impressions have been vague and poorly integrated.

It is preferable to give him, instead of a free field in which to place the pegs, a restricted field which he must organize such as selecting pegs of a given color and arranging them in rows. This will help him to achieve a better integration of the visual and motor aspects of the task.

We speak of integration as the unified functioning of the total organism. The organism functions as a whole. If one of its parts misfunctions, the whole organism tends to misfunction. The activities of perceptual, motor, verbal and conceptual systems are interdependent; each functions in conjunction with the other. It appears that in brain-damaged children, the interaction of these systems is less adequate than in the normal child. As a consequence, the imbalance we speak of becomes manifest.

It is common that one psychologic system, because it may be less damaged, develops more adequately than the others. The disparity is enhanced by the child's natural tendency to use the less damaged system in preference to the damaged one. Thus, children whose verbal-conceptual abilities are better developed than their manual-perceptual ones will tend to talk instead of do. The child with the reverse disparity, good performance but poor verbal abilities, will be very happy to build and construct or practice athletic skills but will avoid participating in activities demanding verbal facility. It is evident that the child's optimum development depends on stimulating the use of the less adequate abilities and so bringing these disparate processes into a more even balance.

When the Other Child reaches the age when his public schooling would normally begin, the parents find themselves at one of the crossroads in the singular life experience of this child. Until this point, the child's deviation from the normal has been masked by the protection of the home. Now, for the first time, the child enters public life, or is expected to. He is required to plunge into a system whose expectations are geared to the developmental profile of the normal child. In such a system, the brain-injured child is likely to fail, for the reason that he is not normal within the definition of most public school systems. We say likely to fail because some brain-injured children manage to adjust to public school.

The paths of learning the educable brain-injured child must travel to achieve an education are only now being blazed. While the problem of mental retardation has been recognized for more than a century in American education, few public school systems recognize brain injury as a specific cause of mental or academic retardation requiring a specific program.

Only rarely is the brain-injured child identified as such in the public school system. His distractibility and perceptual difficulties are regarded as symptoms of immaturity or lack of "readiness" instead of pathologic signs of brain damage. It may be assumed he will somehow grow out of these difficulties. Or it may be assumed that his inability to adjust to the classroom or keep up with normal children are evidences of low intelligence. As a consequence, we frequently find brain-injured children of normal or near normal intelligence in classes for the mentally retarded nonbrain-injured child, or repeating grades in school systems which have no special provisions for children with learning difficulties, or unacceptable to the public school system. In all the states, special programs are provided for physically and mentally handicapped children, but not in all school districts.

The Other Child's anomalous situation with respect to these programs is only now beginning to be recognized. Programs of special education exist for the child who is normal mentally but who physically cannot follow the routines or make use of the facilities provided for children who are physically normal. They exist for children who cannot benefit from instruction because they cannot see or hear as well as others. And they exist for children whose rate of learning is so slow that they require more explanation, more practice and simpler concepts to learn than the average child. There are few provisions for the child who hears and sees normally, who walks, runs, climbs stairs and even rides a bike, and whose ability is close to or within normal limits but who cannot learn.

We regard the best situation for the brain-injured child as the program which recognizes him as brain-injured, which assesses his difficulties in terms of their physiologic origin and which provides a learning program which takes these difficulties into account.

Most primary grade teachers have encountered the child "who couldn't learn." In most respects, except for a certain appearance of vagueness in his eyes, he appeared to be a perfectly normal child. But his behavior was not normal. Sometimes he seemed to be bright and alert. At other times, he seemed to be woodenly dull. He could not color or mark the "things that look alike" in his workbook. He did not learn to read. More disturbing, however, was his behavior. He was hardly ever still. His hyperactivity was a disturbing exaggeration of the wriggling of the six year old. His interest was focused on the children in his vicinity rather than the teacher at the front of the classroom and he would engage in playful poking, blowing, elbowing and other such activities in his desire to form a friendly relationship with the children.

He might get up and walk around the room in the middle of a lesson. He would hum, shuffle his feet or kick them steadily against his desk often listening attentively to the noise they made. When given permission to go to the washroom he might not return and the teacher would find him in conversation with another teacher, the school custodian or just roaming the empty corridor. After he was reprimanded by the teacher he was sincerely and pathetically contrite. But his behavior did not change.

He seemed to be unable to concentrate on anything, yet nothing escaped his attention. He was the one who noticed the loss of a tiny stone in the teacher's brooch and loudly called attention to it. If the classroom flag was moved from its usual position, he was the first to notice it and ask endless questions about it. Occasionally, he might cry or have a tantrum over a trivial disappointment. Sometimes these emotional upsets would occur for no reason apparent to the teacher.

None of the techniques of discipline or teaching the teacher knew had any lasting effect on this child. He was a continual misfit and a disruption to the class. After a while, the child was taken out of school after the school authorities had convinced the parents that the child was not "ready." It was suggested that the child remain at home until he was older or until he could enter a special class for retarded children.

A child who fits this description usually has a perceptual disturbance of some severity. To him the pictures in the workbook all look very much alike and to pick out the ones that are different is a formidable undertaking. The words and pictures on the teacher's reading charts appear to him as marks with no perceptible organization nor meaning. As a result, he turns to that which has meaning for him—the details of his experience which he can organize and comprehend. These may be the open shoelace, the stone in the brooch, the flag which was moved, the child in front of or behind him and so on.

He wanders away from the reading group because its power to attract and hold him there is minimal since its procedures are meaningless to him. Other more meaningful stimuli compete successfully for his attention. The teacher's techniques, no matter how skillful, are ineffectual because they do not reach the core of his difficulty. She is approaching the problem with the assumption that the child's motivation is poor—that he "lacks interest." This is certainly obvious, but it is the result and not the cause. He lacks interest because he lacks the ability to perceive—to organize meaningfully the social structure of the class and the material she is presenting to the rest of the children. Until he can be helped to organize his percepts, his behavior will remain essentially unchanged.

Another brain-injured child who is a great puzzle to the teacher is quite different from the one just described. This child does not have as much difficulty perceiving the classroom social structure or the prereading activities. His worksheets have more errors than those of the other children but they are "passable." His coloring and drawing may not be very good but the teacher regards them as a satisfactory effort.

He does not disrupt the classroom as the earlier child did. In fact, he stays in his seat and does what is expected of all of the children. An observant teacher will note that he appears to be paying attention but it does not have the active, alert quality she would like to see. Often his attention wanders to extraneous objects or he "daydreams." Frequently, his contributions to the class discussions or answers to questions miss the mark—he reports irrelevant happenings or insignificant detail as important.

The realization of this child's problems comes at the end of the first year of school or sometimes not before the second year when it becomes evident that he is not learning. The teacher is baffled because the child is intelligent, his vocabulary is good, his effort was satisfactory, he had no behavior problems to prevent him from learning, yet the instruction she gave successfully to the others did not "take" in his case. Often this child is tutored over the summer or during the school year, hoping that more intensive instruction will correct the difficulty. The results are frequently as discouraging as the classroom experience was.

Why has this child failed? Psychological study usually reveals that this brain-injured child has a very mild or minimal damage affecting several functions. His perceptual disturbance is very slight. In fact, until he had to deal with letters in words he was able to "get by" without being noticeably different. The disturbance is only apparent when he is faced with tasks of some complexity such as are included on a psychological examination or involved in differentiating one or two hundred words from each other.

It is usually also found that his perception and organization of auditory stimuli are poor. He confuses speech sounds which are similar or he may reverse syllables within a word such as "emeny" for "enemy." The damage is often so mild that the child may be without a very obvious speech defect. While his enunciation may not be perfect it is satisfactory enough for him once more to "get by." With a slight visual perceptual disturbance and a slight auditory perceptual disturbance this child had a double handicap to overcome, which was unimportant until these two functions had to work together with great precision in learning academic skills.

Frequently, the child's failure to learn in school is the first indication to the parents that their child is significantly different from other children. Other differences parents may have noticed may have been so slight that they were attributed to the normal variation of children. Such instances have been reported to us so frequently that they appear to form a rather typical experience with many brain-injured children.

Now and then, a teacher attempts to grapple with the problem herself. But without special training in methods of teaching the brain-injured, and without an understanding of the reasons for the child's behavior oddities and inability to learn in the normal classroom, the teacher herself cannot be expected to cope with the problem.

Educators, like other professional people trying earnestly to do their jobs, tend to rely on formalized concepts of education and child development in the application of teaching methods. In the main, it is well that they do so. Otherwise, education would be a chaotic experience. Where the normative educational approach does not recognize the brain-injured child as a special case in education, parents cannot expect the teacher to recognize the specifics of the problem.

Much of the approach to the child in the modern school, we have found, is guided by theories of child behavior which relate to the normal child but not to the Other Child. One of these notions is the concept of "readiness." In general, this term means that by the age of six years the normal child of normal intelligence has matured physiologically and through experience sufficiently to begin to learn reading, writing and numbers. The notion of readiness contains the underlying assumption of normal, balanced growth of the central nervous system. It assumes such growth is universal, and that the rate of development is about the same in all normal children. There is no question that these assumptions rest on a firm foundation of test data and educational experience.

While the concept of "readiness" may apply to the normal child in designating a level of mental development at a particular age, does it apply to the child who is not normal? If readiness is thought to be an expression of neural maturation and experiences, then lack of readiness can be dealt with by giving the organism more time in which to mature neurologically and to accumulate experiences.

In the case of the brain-injured child, we are convinced that the concept of readiness does not apply as fully as it does in the normal child and to attempt to make it apply is a mistake. In our observation, the brain-injured child who is not "ready" to attend public school at the age of six will never be ready in the same sense that the normal child is ready.

The child with a diffuse damage which has affected several psychological systems has been prevented from building into his behavior the learnings which signify readiness in the normal child. All learning depends on previous learning. The brain-injured child's learning has been spotty and unorganized; he has had to spend more than the expected amount of time in grasping simple relationships. He has only a part of the foundation on which to add more complex learnings.

The child with a selective damage, that is, a damage which has affected one psychological system more than another may be "ready" to advance in one area but not in another. If his damage is mainly in visual perception, and his auditory-verbal development has been relatively normal he may be "ready" to learn anything which depends mainly on the use of his unimpaired auditory-verbal abilities, and greatly lacking in readiness to learn skills which would be based on an intact visual perceptual system. In addition, the brain-injured child's perceptual disturbances set up specific barriers to learning which time alone will not remove.

Instead of waiting for growth alone to bring about maturation the brain-injured child needs experiences which will stimulate him to perceive more accurately and in a more related and organized way. The years from six to eight are among the optimum for perceptual development; yet this child, who requires more perceptual training than the normal child, often is required by conventional school systems to wait because he is not "ready."

We do not wish to give the impression that maturation does not produce changes in the perception and behavior of the brain-injured child. It does. It is not yet clear whether these changes come about through actual physiological growth of nervous tissue or whether they result from functional reorganization brought about by learning. The point is that the child may not mature in time to keep in step with the school schedule of normal children.

We have seen that the perceptual functioning of brain-injured children can be improved through appropriate techniques. Therefore, he "grows" perceptually, as measured by tests, at a rate faster than would be expected as a result of physical growth and unspecific learnings.

Another concept presumed to have application to the normal child, is the one called "span of attention." What is "span of attention"? How can "attention" be measured? Let us suppose we can time "span of attention" with a stop watch. Let us consider what we are measuring. We are timing attention. But what is attention? Is it the ability to concentrate? If so, how does one go about timing the period of concentration in another person?

We assume the child is paying attention if he is looking at the teacher and remains passive while the teacher is talking to the class. But is the child actually paying attention? Or could it be that his attention is wandering and that he only appears to be paying attention? As far as the brain-injured child is concerned, the phrase "span of attention" is a negative way of accounting for a positive phenomenon—distractibility. And distractibility is not the failure to pay attention, but the tendency to pay too much attention to too many stimuli. Like "readiness," the phrase "span of attention" is a commonly used term which obscures the real problem of the brain-injured child. If the child's "span of attention" is "too short," how does one go about lengthening it? The teacher who views the problem of the distractible child in these terms is defeated at the outset. But if the teacher regards the child's distractibility in terms of scattered or unselective attention—that is, his tendency to attend to all things at once and to nothing in particular—then a method of dealing with the situation is easy to discern. That is simply to reduce the number of possible stimulus situations likely to distract the child from the lesson. The fact that this approach to the problem of distractibility has a physiologic basis may not be as important to the teacher as the fact that it works in practice.

To deal with the problem successfully, a special learning environment must be created for the child. It is one that differs markedly from the normal classroom environment. This is one of many reasons why at the primary grade level the brain-injured child requires a special class.

Because of the Other Child's tendency to respond to details of a number of stimulus situations, his classroom environment is arranged with the utmost simplicity. The purpose of this arrangement is to protect him from the distractions he is not yet able to ignore.

In such a classroom, the windows may be curtained or painted out. A pleasant diffuse light comes through, but the child is not attracted by what is going on outside. Neither procedure is necessary if the windows do not face the street or if the classroom is on an upper floor. The child's desk faces the wall so that he is not distracted by other children in the room.

There are no decorations on the wall to intrude into his perceptual field. Except for essential furniture the classroom is as bare as a classroom can be. The teacher dresses plainly, without ornamentation. Interruptions from the outside are held at the minimum. In this way, a therapeutic environment is created for the Other Child. Its structure is easy for him to grasp. Along with it, he comes into a quiet, steady routine. The number of children in the room, including him, does not exceed eight. In such an environment, the child's distractions are reduced to the minimum.

Another kind of distractibility which is commonly seen is what might be termed conceptual distractibility, or an interruption of a trend of thought by wayward associations only loosely related to the trend. For example, in reading about a dog, the child may be impelled to think of Rin-Tin-Tin, the Wonder Dog, and asks, "What is a wonder?" Or, the sound of the verb, "does," triggers the association of "Duz, a miracle for clothes," and he asks, "What is a miracle?"

Some children appear to be day dreaming while a lesson is being explained or an assignment is being given. But the content of the day dreaming has none of the organized fantasy or emotional coloring of the child seeking to escape from reality. This child will usually be found having difficulty grasping the organization of the lesson or assignment, keeping sequences in order, or abstracting essential features.

The approach, as in the case of the child who is perceptually distractible, is to simplify the conceptual task so that the child can understand it or to simplify and clarify the terms in which the task is explained.

But removing distractions is only setting the stage so that the child will be responsive to the teacher's instruction. The next step is to provide him with lessons, or learning experiences. These will help him to master skills which the normal child has acquired even before entering school. However, before much effective learning can occur, the child must be able to organize his lessons, as well as his wider classroom environment, into a coherent structure. To do this it is necessary that his tasks be simple enough to insure success but so designed that they will lead him to a better organized performance than he was capable of before the task.

A child who has never been able to trace pictures in children's coloring books (because he could not organize the lines into a meaningful pattern) can trace short colored lines through onion skin or draw a crayon line from dot to dot across a page. On this simple level the child can begin to organize the kind of perceptual-motor experiences which are directly pertinent to academic achievement.

The learning tasks should always be so planned that their pattern is perceptible to the child. He himself should be able to decide where to begin, when the task is complete, and whether he has accomplished it reasonably satisfactorily. In attempting tasks which are too complex for him the Other Child is often confused and at a loss to decide these basic things. He depends on the teacher to organize the task for him, asking her to tell him where he should begin, whether he is all through, and whether it is well done. The often heard, well meaning reply, "That's quite good but tomorrow I think you can do even better" neither encourages nor helps the child. He cannot know how to do better if he does not know wherein he failed to do well. On a simple task the error is also simple. It can be brought to the child's attention so that tomorrow, or even better, right at the moment it is being discussed he can correct it.

Since the child quickly exhausts the stimulus possibilities of an activity and his attention then scatters to other things, the duration of each task is brief. It may last only a minute or two. But a lesson period consists of a series of short tasks, each planned so that they can be organized by the child, executed successfully and recognized as completed.

In this way the child gains confidence in his ability to achieve and is encouraged to attempt more and more. He also develops invaluable habits of completing what he begins and of correcting errors which he himself discovers or which are brought to his attention.

In other terms, the teacher has provided him with a stimulus situation which is clear and simple enough for him to organize. He responds to his percept of it with some motor activity, thus stimulating perceptual-motor integration, and the task provides the feedback to tell him whether his percept of it was correct or not. There are many such activities for the child to do, all of which require that he perceive correctly the forms in his visual environment and that he organize their relationships to each other.

It is easier for most brain-injured children to copy a pattern produced by someone else than to originate it themselves. In order to produce a pattern or a form, one needs first to have organized other patterns and to have learned what "form" means.

The child cannot "create" or "express" himself adequately until he has first taken in organized experiences which are then recombined to create a new structure. Many of the child's classroom experiences are designed with this in view. In the beginning the child builds patterns which the teacher has made with peg boards, cube blocks and blocks of different shapes. He learns how the blocks are combined to form a pattern of colors or how their different shapes can be put together to make a larger form. In this way he learns to organize a figure against a background, and to select a part out of this whole figure for particular attention. Gradually he is expected to build simple organized structures of his own.

The teaching of other perceptual-motor skills is comparable. The child is shown by the material or the task itself how to organize his percepts. Gradually less structure is built into the task and more is required from the child. The brain-injured child who cannot color within lines may be given a stencil in the form of a cardboard with a square cut-out. He then colors within the square when the cardboard is placed over a piece of paper. In this way he learns to perceive, through the structure of the task, the correct end product of his coloring and the technique by which it is achieved. Later, he colors a square formed by heavy black lines and still later a figure outlined in narrower lines.

Two things are accomplished by such a program. The young brain-injured child develops two aspects of "readiness": He learns to persist at a task until it is completed and he begins to differentiate forms and their relationships in preparation for the serious business of reading and computation. For the somewhat older brain-injured child a whole new world is often opened—a world of forms and patterns which he had formerly disregarded as being so complicated and difficult that it was for others but not for him. Often such a child will begin for the first time to make puzzles, draw or construct with blocks during his leisure time.

What becomes of the child with the "limited span of attention" in this kind of class? In the environment we have described, we find that the so-called "span of attention" has miraculously increased in a few short weeks. The child has become able to focus his attention on the task placed before him. He no longer keeps shifting his attention all over the room. There is really no miracle involved in the transformation. Once the child has been able to organize his classroom experience and begins to derive satisfaction from the achievement of even simple tasks, he finds the classroom a comfortable place to be and relates himself actively to the learning process. External distractions no longer have the power to disrupt the perceptual organization required in the performance of the task.

The child has achieved a firmer structuring of the task and an improved ability to perceive the relationship between it and other stimuli. He may be distracted momentarily by some external event, but he is able quickly to relegate it into the background of his total awareness and return to the work he is doing.

As he progresses in this way and becomes able to integrate an increasing number of stimulus situations into meaningful patterns, the necessity for such careful control of the classroom environment diminishes. He can now be seated in the more conventional classroom arrangement and various display or teaching materials can be used as fully as the teacher wishes. All of these arrangements, however, have as one of their goals the ultimate mastery of the academic tools so that the child can resume his place in the mainstream of school life. How does the child's brain injury affect this goal?

The learning of academic skills is believed to rest on a number of psychological processes which can be identified. For example, to master the first step in reading—identifying words—the child must have an adequate vocabulary development and must be able visually to differentiate forms, recognize differences in direction of visually presented figures and organize several forms spatially in a given relationship to one another. He must be able to direct his attention to a given perceptual pattern according to an arbitrary sequence (from left to right and from top to bottom). If the words he reads occur in a sentence in a beginning reading book, he must be able to quickly and easily organize them into figure and ground in an unvarying sequence, each word becoming for the moment it is read a figure, and dropping immediately to the status of background as the next word emerges into the foreground.

But reading is not only dependent on knowledge of word meanings and the ability to visually identify shapes. It depends heavily on skill in decoding visually presented figures into auditory-verbal units. To do this accurately the child must have developed an auditory-perceptual organization comparable to the visual-perceptual one just described. He must be aware, not only of the meanings of the words he hears, but of their phonetic characteristics. The word sounds he hears must have "form" to him—they must be identifiable as characteristically distinct from other word sounds. He must, furthermore, be aware of the temporal organization of the various parts of a word sound, that is, the sequence in which they are uttered.

During the process of learning to read, these two psychological systems—the auditory and visual—must work together in an impressively precise relationship. The visual input to the organism must be highly accurate and must enter in an orderly temporal sequence. It must then be "matched" to appropriate speech sounds which, when combined, will be recognized as words communicating meaning. The brain-injured child may experience difficulty at any point in this very complex process.

If his visual perceptual ability is disturbed, letter or word shapes may appear similar to him, or if his directional orientation is not well established he will confuse the ones which differ mainly in this characteristic. If his perception of spatial relationships is poor, words which differ in the order and arrangement of letters as "split" and "spilt" will be confused. If he has difficulty maintaining stable figure-ground relations, he will read erratically, skipping words, and lines, and being distracted by the pictures.

A child whose auditory perception is impaired may not detect differences in sounds which are quite similar such as short a and e, ch, sh, and so on. If temporal organization is poor he will tend to transpose sounds or syllables in words as "deks" for "desk," "bisghetti" for "spaghetti," etc. He may experience difficulty in combining two or three sounds, spoken separately, into a word.

The program for the brain-injured child is planned to take into account the possibility that any of these confusions may occur. Instruction is given even before he begins to read to help the child to be able to make the discriminations and organizations which are required. Therefore, he matches many different shapes among which are letter shapes and learns to be alert to sequence by building words from letters.

In order to sharpen auditory awareness the children are given "listening" training in small groups. They listen attentively to whether two words are alike or different in sound, whether they begin or end with the same sounds, or whether they have the same vowel sound. For individual work the children sort out or draw pictures of things which begin with the same sound. They begin the process of auditory analysis by identifying parts of words which sound alike.

Finally, the visual and auditory processes are combined. Whatever assistance or crutch the child may need in order to function in spite of his disabilities is freely given to him. If the auditory side of this associative process is weak, and he "forgets" the sounds for various letters he may need to have a dictionary of sounds, or a key, to which he may refer at any time he needs it. He may need to read word cards on which the consonant and vowel combinations are drawn in different colors to remind him of the necessity for matching accurately what he sees with what he says. If he is very distractible or fatigues quickly, he may read separate sentences on cards or separate pages from a reader cut up and mounted for this purpose. If he can write well, it will help him to form the associations between sight and sound by having him write the words he studies, saying them as he writes. When he actually begins the process of reading in a book, if he is distracted by the pictures or heedless of small words and punctuation marks, he may need to have a cardboard mask covering the page so that only one or a few words are in view at a time.

The process of learning arithmetic is approached in a similar manner. There is evidence to suggest that the learning of computation skills rests on the development of a visual spatial scheme in which quantities are seen in relation to one another. To do this the child must again be able to organize a figure against a background and to accurately compare one quantity with another in respect to size and position in a series. He must be able to shift foreground and background at will, turning his attention from the whole to the parts which compose it or from two lesser parts to the greater whole which results from their combination. Finally, after he has organized quantities in relation to one another in ways which are directly perceptible to him, he must begin to carry in his imagery some kind of representation of these relationships.

The same activities which help to develop form perception and figure-ground organization as a basis for reading serve to prepare the child for arithmetic as well. In addition to these activities he is given many more specific ones which pertain directly to the learning of arithmetic. All of the elementary processes are practiced with concrete aids. These are so designed that they will provide a good scheme which can be kept in mind as an image when the time comes to discard the device. When the child knows the number sequence and can count, he begins to organize groups into patterns such as those seen on dominoes. These patterns he matches, builds on pegboards, draws, pastes from squares of colored paper, and so on. From this perception of groups he goes on to see the same quantities as lengths, and then to an abacus—a number device with rows of beads, each row containing 10 beads—which he uses for computation. Again, at any point along the way, if the child's performance is hindered by the disabilities created by his organic damage he is given a crutch or an aid to relieve the problem until the time when he can successfully perform the mental activity required.

Some children lose their place in working a page of problems because of these difficulties in figure-ground organization. Such a child may be taught to underline each number in red pencil as he puts the corresponding quantity on the abacus in order to keep his place. Another child may not be able to visualize the abacus in order to do his arithmetic without a concrete aid, and may need to sketch it as a series of lines which he can then use to solve his problems.

In teaching any of the academic subjects, the teaching method and materials are adapted to circumvent the disabilities arising from the child's brain damage. If the child is easily distracted (and distractions occur more easily when the organization of a stimulus situation is weak), he is not taught in a group or by the teacher's demonstration at the front of the class. Instead, the teacher seats herself by the child's desk and makes certain that she has his attention before giving her explanation or demonstration. The greater the space between teacher and child, the stronger the likelihood that it will be occupied with irrelevant stimuli.

Because of the child's difficulty in figure-ground organization he is confused by having much material on a page. Therefore, he may have only a few problems on a page or a few words to match or read. Different colors are used to help him to keep his place easily. Also, because of his distractibility it is preferable to give him only what he will need for the completion of a lesson. A whole book or workbook may be too stimulating and may induce him to leaf through its pages to look at the pictures. An entire box of crayons may lead to playing with them or trying out their colors; he will be better served by having only the one or two colors he may need.

The child with a visual-perceptual disturbance will organize small wholes meaningfully, that is, he will respond to details, and will tend to neglect the larger whole of which the detail may form a part. Teaching by selecting large wholes for study asks the child to depend on the very ability in which he is deficient. He will learn to read more readily if he learns the auditory equivalent of the details—the letters or groups of letters rather than the whole words. Consequently, brain-injured children usually progress better in reading if taught by phonics—a system which teaches small units—rather than by the whole word system which requires the ability to retain and analyze large units.

It is characteristic for brain-injured children to have difficulty in seeing relationships and in drawing conclusions based on these relationships. They do not abstract meaning well from a given set of stimuli. Therefore, the teaching method does not rely on the child's ability to make generalizations or see relationships. Instead, the teacher will lead the child to or actually point out the relationships, assisting the child in this way to perceive the given stimuli as normal persons do.

The teacher uses whatever area of proficiency the child may have to achieve a meaningful organization, or percept, of the task. If the child shows a good ability to verbalize but is poor perceptually, the teacher may use verbal explanation to aid the child in coming to an organized visual percept. The child himself may gradually develop this into a detour technique. Such a child may "talk to himself" about a task, organizing it in verbal terms, saying "here's a red block in the corner, then a yellow block," etc. In learning to write he may instruct himself to "go up, then down, now put a cross on it," while making a "t."

If a child's kinesthetic organization is relatively good, it can be used in teaching him to write and to associate the sounds to letters or words. He can be taught the form of a letter by correctly organizing, then recalling, the movement pattern which is characteristic for that letter. At the chalkboard, the teacher may guide his arm through the required motions, making it as large as the child's arm will allow or she may guide the child in writing the letter in a flat pan of modeling clay. At the same time, the child says the phonetic equivalent (the "sound") of the visual or kinesthetic letter pattern he is making.

To a child who is able to think abstractly, the teacher would point out all of the relationships in a task. Such a child profits by being taught rules like "any number multiplied by five will end in either zero or five." He is more likely to remember the answer to 4 times 8 as double the answer to 4 times 4 than as a rote association.

Teaching by means of, or through the strongest abilities, however, does not mean that the child is thus excused from using his damaged abilities. A skill which requires the interaction of more than one mental faculty cannot be built if one of the faculties is not functioning. The semblance of such a skill can be acquired but it is like a house of cards—likely to tumble from a weight it cannot bear.

A child with poor auditory discrimination and analysis may learn to read by sight—by associating the word name to the visual form of the word. A child with a good rote memory may learn number combinations without being able to visualize the quantities they represent. In either case, the road leads to a blind alley. It brings the learner to a halt, unable to progress because he has taken a side spur rather than the main track.

To keep the child on the course which will eventually lead him to the goal achieved by the normal child, it is necessary that he use every faculty required for the mastery of a given skill, even though some faculties may be weak or inefficient. To do this he needs all the support that can be given by crutches, the particular aids and approaches that the teacher can devise.

It cannot be taken for granted that he will use his damaged ability however, as it may be easier for him to attempt some other approach. Therefore, the teaching method or the task needs to be so designed that the child will make an effort to learn through the integration of good and poor abilities and not avoid what may be a difficult task for him. This is important for the teacher to keep in mind in evaluating a child's success. A success based on the use of an inefficient method (as finger-counting in arithmetic) or on some peripheral clue (memory for single letters in reading) is a compromise rather than a real success. The teacher's problem will be to substitute an approach which will require revision of the child's method.

Obviously, if the child is being asked to use his disabled abilities he will benefit from exercising them. With this in mind the child is given, as part of his school assignment, numerous activities dependent on a given ability for their completion. Some of these activities are games, some are formal lessons. To stimulate the use of visual-perceptual abilities, the child continues on a more advanced level the activities mentioned earlier for developing readiness—he builds puzzles, constructs block and peg designs, and so on. He is taught to play checkers, dominoes and various table games. Children with auditory-perceptual problems have, in addition to their group experiences, lessons to do at their desks to give further practice in distinguishing sounds in words. In this way the child progresses to a mastery of the basic academic skills and ultimately to the acquisition of as much knowledge as his interests and general abilities permit.

As the child learns to adjust to the special class, he can be given a part of his instruction in regular classes at the grade level in which he can perform satisfactorily. In this way, he can be integrated into the life of the public school. Such a program follows the principle of integrating rather than isolating the child. But the integration must proceed under careful supervision. As it succeeds, the need for supervision recedes.

For some brain-injured children, a private residential school may be indicated as the most effective therapy. The process of integrating the child into the public school special or regular class must necessarily be postponed until the child is deemed ready to make the transition. When he is ready to make it, parents and teachers should recognize that the child requires special help in orienting himself to a new environment.

Once adjusted to the public school classroom situation, many brain-injured children become adequate students and make a reasonably good adjustment to their age group. We frequently see the child who has been such a severe behavior problem in the first grade that he cannot be tolerated in the normal classroom transformed into a diligent, earnest pupil after several years of effective special education.

We have been discussing what we consider to be a practical approach to the education of the brain-injured child who is educable. We cannot overemphasize the basis of this approach: one which identifies his learning and behavioral difficulties and which provides the environment and program to deal specifically with them.

How workable is this approach in a public school system? The answer may be indicated by the experience of the Joliet, Illinois grade school district where a special class for brain-injured children was established in 1950 and a second one in 1955.

Joliet is an industrial city of 50,000 on the Illinois Waterway about 30 miles southwest of Chicago. Its school system might be considered average for a small, midwestern city. The city and its environs are served by two school districts, each a separate administrative and taxing unit. One is the grade school district and the other is the high school district. In 1949, the Illinois Department of Public Instruction selected the Joliet grade school district as the site of an experimental class for brain-injured children. The origin of this experiment is related to the work of the Cove Schools for Brain-Injured Children at Racine, Wisconsin and Evanston, Illinois.

Psychologists in the state office of public instruction had become concerned about a number of children in classes for the educable mentally handicapped who showed the learning difficulties and behavioral characteristics of the brain-injured child. It was reasoned that a special educational program along the lines of the one developed by the Cove Schools might accelerate the learning of children who proved to be educational misfits because of brain injury. The state office selected an experienced teacher in special education and arranged for her to take training in the teaching of brain-injured children at the Cove Schools for one year as preparation for teaching the special class in Joliet.

The Joliet grade school district superintendent and board of trustees were receptive to the idea. The state paid the salary of the teacher and in addition reimbursed the school district at the rate of $300 a child a year under the state program for the physically and mentally handicapped. The school district furnished the classroom and handled the administrative details of determining eligibility, arranging transportation for children who lived outside of the area normally served by the school and aligning the class in the total school program.

There were several reasons for selecting Joliet as the site for the experiment. One was the willingness of school officials to participate. Another was the availability of a qualified psychologist in Joliet to assist in the program. Joliet had a well established program for the educable mentally handicapped from which the brain-injured children could be selected for the experiment. Also, the city was close enough to Chicago so that the children would not have to travel far for medical and psychological examinations at the University of Illinois Medical Center on Chicago's west side.

The plan was to select ten children, from six to ten years old, for the class. The children were determined as being brain-injured by psychological and neurological examination. Two control classes were set up as a basis on which to compare the academic progress of the brain-injured children in the experimental class with that of brain-injured children and retarded children who were not brain-injured in the classes for the educable mentally handicapped.

The control classes had to be dropped from the experiment as "controls," however, because in each a number of the children moved away and unavoidable changes in teaching personnel took place. Consequently, the special class for the brain-injured became a demonstration class, rather than an experimental one.

In the neurological examinations of the children, the school authorities in Joliet ran into the same ambiguity which parents of brain-injured children have encountered in attempting to get a medical diagnosis spelling out brain damage. Some of the children did not display neurological symptoms of brain damage. In several cases, the electroencephalograph gave no positive indication. This is not unusual, as we have observed.

Clinical evidence of brain damage which is confined to the higher processes of perception, concept formation and reasoning shows up more clearly in psychological testing than in medical examination. Often, it does not show up at all in a neurologic examination or on the electroencephalograph, a machine for measuring the electrical output of the brain. In cases in which the medical evidence was ambiguous, the evidence of the psychological tests was adopted if it showed the typical behavioral responses of brain injury.

The class was located at the Cunningham School in Joliet, in a hilltop neighborhood of modest frame houses, rather typical of the middle income residential section of a midwestern city. Before opening the class, school authorities, the school principal and the teacher carried out a carefully planned program of education for the benefit of the school staff and the community.

The Parent-Teacher Association was briefed on the purposes of the class. School authorities felt it was important to stress the fact that the class was serving the entire city, not simply the pupils of the Cunningham School. This was done to allay any gossip that there was such a concentration of brain-injured children in the Cunningham School that a special room had to be set aside for them. Also stressed was the notion that Joliet had been especially privileged in being selected by the state office as the site of the demonstration.

The project was discussed at the first teachers' meeting at the Cunningham School. The principal made it clear that some of the children in the special class eventually would be tried in regular classes at the school and urged the teachers to become familiar with the program and the problem it was designed to solve. Parents of the children selected for the class were given a detailed explanation of what the demonstration class was trying to do. Joliet authorities anticipated that it was not enough to create such a class; the community and the teachers had to be sold on it in advance.

Historically, the significance of the class as a milestone in public education can hardly be overstated. It appears to have been the first public school class specifically for brain-injured children in the United States. The teaching method for the class followed essentially the principles as outlined earlier in the chapter.

The purpose of the program was to rehabilitate brain-injured children to the point at which they could take their places in the educational process—in a regular grade, a special class for the physically handicapped or a special class for the educable mentally handicapped. Thus, education becomes a treatment process.

In many respects, the special class was "special" indeed compared to all the other classes in the Joliet grade school district. Visitors were immediately struck by the appearance of the classroom. Instead of the lively colors lent by displays of art creations of the pupils and the variety of materials in the ordinary classroom, this one had a subdued and spaciously uncluttered quality.

The lower half of the windows were painted with opaque paint, admitting light, but preventing the children from seeing out. Each child's desk faced the wall. Screens were available for each child whose distractibility did not yield to the previous measures. Cupboards were kept closed. All pictures and bulletin boards were removed to create a nondistracting uniformity of background.

The teaching procedures were based on the principle that the child's learning handicaps had to be mitigated or circumvented before he could learn. Three years after the class opened its doors, the academic progress of the ten brain-injured children was evaluated as well as their intellectual and social growth.

In comparison to the experience of brain-injured children in classes for the educable mentally handicapped, the academic progress of the ten in the demonstration class over three years was remarkable. Four of the children progressed one year in academic achievement for each year spent in the demonstration class, thus making the same rate of progress as the normal child in the regular class.

Four others gained about two and one-half years over the three-year period (or one and one-half years over a two-year period). This represents a definite acceleration over the usual progress made by educable mentally handicapped pupils, according to the report of the state department psychologist. One pupil achieved at the rate of two years over the three-year period and one made one year of progress in two years. One year of progress in two years is about the rate of progress by children in the educable mentally handicapped program, according to the report.

In summary, 90 per cent of the group showed a higher rate of progress than the average for the educable mentally handicapped program and 10 per cent equalled that rate. But even more astonishing was the fact that 40 per cent progressed at the same rate as the normal child in the regular class. These children were thus enabled to take their places in regular classes.

In the area of intellectual functioning, measurement appeared somewhat ambiguous. Only one child made significant improvement on one well known and widely used test of intelligence. On another equally well known test, however, four children made important gains in the functioning level of intelligence. Indeed, two of them progressed enough that they could no longer be considered mentally handicapped.

All ten children showed improvement in the area of social adjustment. They became less impulsive. Their hyperactivity decreased. Their ability to look at the world realistically increased. Seven made noticeable improvement in their degree of independence. Eight showed improvement in social relationships. In this area, one made no noticeable improvement and one seemed to become more withdrawn.

As a result of the demonstration class, five of the ten were recommended for placement in a regular grade on the basis of academic achievement, social adjustment and a trial placement in a regular grade. Three were recommended for educable mentally handicapped classes, although two of them showed the potential for eventual placement in a regular grade. Two were retained in the demonstration class for further training, but one showed a potential for later placement in a regular grade. All five children who were placed in regular grades in the fall of 1954 had continued their academic progress at the normal rate.

The success of the demonstration class for brain-injured children in Joliet led to the establishment of a second class for brain-injured children of normal intelligence.

The Illinois Department of Public Instruction has been wary about proclaiming the success of the demonstration. One reason is that such a program is limited by the number of teachers with adequate training to take a class, and they are few. Another reason was the failure of the demonstration—by academic standards—to qualify as an experiment. Critics could always point to the lack of controls, which, as we have related, broke down early because of the shifting of teachers and pupils in the control classes.

We place emphasis on two aspects of the education of the brain-injured child who is educable. One is a program of preschool training in nursery school or kindergarten to develop his social awareness. The other is his primary education in a special class where his disabilities are taken into account.

It is obvious that this job falls on the shoulders of the parents, and that in many instances they must tackle it without community support. But we have seen a whole generation of brain-injured children growing up, and we know that the task of providing the educable child with the kind of training and education he needs holds great rewards for the parents and the child.

For the brain-injured child is a human being who is struggling to adjust to and assert himself in the world under a tremendous handicap. His potential is often greater than it seems, but his handicap is great, too.

His own efforts must not be discounted, for he, too, is battling against his handicap. Given proper help and direction many of these children can live a normal, useful life. That is the measure of victory of the human spirit over odds that at the outset may appear overwhelming.

Index

Autism